The World's Best Kept

Health Secret
REVEALED

By The Leading Wellness Experts

Dr. CJ Mertz
and Leading Wellness Co-Authors

The World's Best Kept Health Secret Revealed/Mertz and Co-Authors

ISBN 0-9744857-0-5

   1. Self-Help   I. The World's Best Kept Health Secret Revealed

Cover Design by Steve Lisi
Book Layout/Design by Clark Kidman
Editing by Jo Ridgway

Chiropractic Press books are available for distribution by emailing info@chiropracticpress.com or calling 715-868-1109.

Attention: Doctors of Chiropractic.
Are you a doctor of chiropractic who would like to become a published best selling author? If so, contact Chiropractic Press, Inc. at 715-868-1109 or email info@chiropracticpress.com for the free special report, "How To Instantly Increase Your Professional Status – Stop Justifying Your Chiropractic Services – And Double Your Practice . . ."

PLEASE READ THIS
DISCLAIMER CAREFULLY

INDEMNITY.

You agree to defend, indemnify, and hold Chiropractic Press, Inc., its officers, directors, employees, agents, licensors, licensees, contributing authors/experts and suppliers, harmless from and against any claims, actions or demands, liabilities and settlements including without limitation, reasonable legal and accounting fees, resulting from, or alleged to result from, your violation of this Disclaimer.

GENERAL.

Chiropractic Press, Inc. is based in the United States of America. Chiropractic Press, Inc. and "Group" make no claims that the Book or the content is appropriate or may be used outside of the United States. Access to the content may not be legal by certain persons or in certain countries. If you access this Book or the content from outside the United States, you do so at your own risk and are responsible for compliance with the laws of your jurisdiction. The following provisions survive the expiration or termination of this Disclaimer for any reason whatsoever: Liability, Indemnity, Jurisdiction, and Complete Agreement.

JURISDICTION.

You expressly agree that exclusive jurisdiction for any dispute with Chiropractic Press, Inc. or "Group", or In any way relating to your use of this Book or content, resides in the courts of the State of Minnesota, United States of America, or it can be moved to a court and jurisdiction of Chiropractic Press, Inc.'s choice. You further agree and expressly consent to the exercise of personal jurisdiction in the courts of the State of Minnesota or a court and jurisdiction of Chiropractic Press, Inc.'s choice in connection with any such dispute including any claim involving Chiropractic Press, Inc. or its contributing experts, licensors, licensees, agents, affiliates, subsidiaries, employees, contractors, officers, directors and content providers.

The terms and conditions of this Disclaimer are governed by the internal substantive laws of the State of Minnesota, without respect to its conflict of law principles and can be moved to a court and jurisdication of Chiropractic Press, Inc's choice and approval. If any provision of this Disclaimer is found to be invalid by any court having competent jurisdiction, the invalidity of such provision shall not affect the validity of the remaining provisions of this Disclaimer, which shall remain in full force and effect. No waiver of any of this Disclaimer shall be deemed a further or continuing waiver of such term or condition or any other term or condition.

COMPLETE AGREEMENT.

This Disclaimer constitutes the entire agreement between you, Chiropractic Press, Inc. and "Group" with respect to the use of this Book and content.

If you do not wish to be bound by this disclaimer, please return this Book to the person who gave you this Book or the place you purchased it for a refund!

CONTENTS

Introduction
Dr. Terry Rondberg

Chapter 1
The World's Best Kept Health Secret Revealed To You

Chapter 2
Could Subluxation Be Hurting You?

Chapter 3
Can Children Have Subluxation?

Chapter 4
The Science of Subluxations

Chapter 5
The Dramatic Difference When Subluxations are Removed

Chapter 6
How To Protect Your Family

Chapter 7
The Healing of Unique Subluxations

INTRODUCTION

❧

By Dr. Terry A. Rondberg, D.C.

There's no doubt that we're undergoing a health care revolution today. People are taking responsibility for their own health more than ever before. They're discarding outmoded medical concepts of treating symptoms and disease, in favor of a wellness approach that encompasses physical, emotional, and spiritual well-being.

Chiropractic is a complex discipline that respects the body's innate self healing ability and can assist the body, often preventing the need for dangerous drugs or invasive surgery.

Few people know as much about chiropractic as Dr. CJ Mertz and even fewer have been able to tell the chiropractic story with such clarity and precision. In this book, he and his colleagues, who are renowned wellness experts, provide readers with a wealth of knowledge that will help them lead healthier, happier – and longer lives.

The material manages to find that delicate balance between technical details and personal narrative that makes chiropractic accessible and understandable. Best of all, this book provides practical tips that readers can use in their daily lives to increase their own health and the wellness of their families. This book presents an incredible opportunity to begin a journey into wellness!

As President of the World Chiropractic Alliance, I have had the honor of knowing CJ for many years. I absolutely believe this may be one of the most important books you will ever read. I encourage everyone interested in true wellness to read it and share it with their friends.

Dr. Terry A. Rondberg, D.C.
President, World Chiropractic Alliance
Publisher, *The Chiropractic Journal*
CEO, Chiropractic Benefit Services

CHAPTER ONE

THE WORLD'S BEST KEPT HEALTH SECRET REVEALED TO YOU

PART ONE

DEFINING WELLNESSCARE

By Dr. CJ Mertz

"Education is the most powerful weapon which you can use to change the world." – Nelson Mandela

It is hard to believe only a few centuries ago, people thought the world was flat. Today, global relationships, travel and commerce enrich our planet. We take our global lifestyles and opportunities for granted as if life has always been this way.

Centuries ago, the "flat world" belief was a matter of life and death. Fortunately, Christopher Columbus didn't hold this belief and set out to discover the new world. By doing so, he changed existence for everyone.

Was the world flat and turned round? Or was the world always round and we hadn't realized it?

Upon the once radical discovery that the world was round, not everyone believed it— even after the evidence proved it to be true. Now we look back with awkward grins and try to imagine how anybody could have thought the world was flat.

Healthcare from Flat to Round

Right now, healthcare and wellnesscare are going through this exact paradigm shift. As of this writing, the term "wellnesscare" can't be found in the dictionary. That is because wellnesscare hasn't been defined…until now.

Several leading health and business experts are predicting

wellnesscare to be America's next trillion-dollar industry.

In North America, along with most of the world, I feel we don't have "healthcare." Our healthcare is actually "sickcare." That is, we focus on ridding our bodies of our sicknesses versus instilling wellness. People have accepted the limited belief that health is defined as a lack of symptoms.

If you aren't sick, then you must be healthy. If you aren't in pain, then you must be healthy. If you aren't tired, then you must be healthy. And, if you are sick, your illness or injury must have been caused from outside yourself and worked its way into your body.

Sickcare, Healthcare and Wellnesscare…The Life Saving Differences

Would you take medicine if you were not sick? What do you suppose would happen if you gave a healthy person medication? You're right. They might just get sick!

There are times sickcare medicine uses a "wait-and-see" approach. What does this mean? When you are sick and go to a sickcare physician, you'll probably receive a battery of tests, a diagnosis and a prescription.

If your condition appears to improve, you will not see your doctor until you get sick again.

If your condition does not improve, you undergo more testing. Your sickcare medical professional may modify or change your diagnosis. You may be asked to try additional or different medications. If your condition persists, you may be asked to consider surgery to remove some dysfunctional part of your body.

It is my belief healthy people rarely get sick. Unhealthy people could be prone to sickness for life.

People hope to avoid strokes, heart attacks or cancers. But, their lifestyle choices could be heading straight in this direction.

People hope they won't suffer from infections, osteoarthritis, osteoporosis, high blood pressure, diabetes and a host of other conditions. They hope their children won't be labeled with ADD, asthma, allergies or worse.

The truth is most hardworking and honest people today simply use "hope management" instead of creating wellness in their lives.

Your family deserves better answers and your future depends upon it.

How Long Has Sickcare Been "The Answer?"

George Washington was the first president of the United States in the 1700's. When he fell ill, he had the best sickcare money could buy. President Washington was diagnosed with toxicity of the blood (bad blood.) The treatment he received included the use of leaches, which were placed on his body to suck out the bad blood. George Washington died during treatment.

You and I would consider this type of treatment barbaric. We couldn't imagine something so gruesome happening to us or anyone we know today.

Looking forward fifty years from now, I believe we could look back on today's use of antibiotics to care for humans as barbaric.

How Could This Be So?

Today, because of the widespread use of antibiotics in "sickcare," we have created strains of bacteria completely antibiotic resistant. Bacteria have grown so powerful they can eat antibiotics like food.

I believe we are moving from sickcare, where we treat illnesses with answers from outside our bodies, to wellnesscare, where we work with the power of the body to heal.

If someone has pain and turns to sickcare for answers, he or she is given a painkiller.

If they have swelling, an anti-inflammatory.

Infection, antibiotic.
High blood pressure, high blood pressure medication.
Muscle spasms, muscle relaxers.
Cramping, cramping medication.
Sinus problems, sinus medication.
Allergies, allergy medication.
Sleeping problems, sleeping medication.
Digestion problems, digestion medication.
Infertility, infertility drugs.
Moodiness, moodiness medication.
Bowel movement problems, bowel movement medication.
This sickcare list can go on indefinitely!

Is Sickcare Medicating Us to Death?

As we age, the belief is our bodies "naturally" breakdown requiring more interventions of medicine. The average American senior citizen ingests multiple prescriptions daily.

There is no doctor in the world who can tell us exactly how all these medications react with each other once they enter *each* individual person's body.

The biggest tragedy however has fallen upon our children, some who endure medications and side effects for lifetimes.

Have children's bodies ever been deficient in behavioral medication? Painkillers? Antibiotics? Of course, NOT! Yet we continue to pour billions of dollars of medications into their bodies, even though many of us believe (and even know) medications are not always the answer.

I believe the "flat world" society of sickcare is coming to an end...and not a moment too soon.

We must embrace the new frontier of wellnesscare with the same boldness used to claim our round world.

I believe healing does not happen from outside-in. Rather it occurs from inside-out.

Many families subscribe to the art, science and philosophy

of wellnesscare. They are living healthy, happy and productive lives as a result.

The Central Operating System for Wellness in Your Body

Physical, mental and emotional well-being requires your mind, body and spirit to co-orchestrate thousands of daily functions to live.

Found within your nervous system is the most sophisticated intelligence network on earth. Mental impulses, generated from within your brain, are transmitted through a half-inch cable known as your spinal cord.

Inside your spinal cord, these brain messages are carried via electrical impulses along a multitude of fiber-optic-like nerves. Your naturally inborn intelligence is so powerful that it is capable of simultaneously directing and monitoring all functions and systems of your body.

Your Body Functioning 100% Healthy

A state of 100% wellness requires the electrical impulses from your brain to travel through your spinal cord and communicate with the right places in your body at the right times.

Think of the volume of communications happening between your brain and body right now. As you read…your body performs what could be called miracles!

You breathe without asking for a breath. Your heart pumps blood to areas of your body you might not even realize you have or need to live. Your body digests food you ate hours ago… and you probably even forgot about after comforted by a full stomach.

Your body functions and creates miracles each moment of your life. Most of us don't notice — until the miracles cease. Illness is when your body is not properly functioning.

The sickcare paradigm may see people as chemical warehouses. In part, they are right. There is chemical imbalance associated with virtually every state of diagnosed lowered health.

The sickcare philosophy includes adding chemicals into a sick body with the goal of trying to regain a normal chemical balance within the body. This could keep people taking chemical medications for weeks, months, years and even lifetimes.

A more natural approach is to locate and remove interferences blocking your brain's communication to your body through your spinal cord information highway. This could allow your brain to send the electrical messages to the cells and parts of your body requiring instruction on how to function properly.

When your instructions are correctly received by your body this could stimulate a perfect sequence of chemical reactions and wellness.

When it comes to healing, chemical medications pumped into your body are not always the answer...and certainly not my choice. I have found that the body needs interference removed from its spinal cord and nervous system so natural innate intelligence can communicate healthy functioning messages to cells and body parts.

The Wellnesscare Revolution

Chiropractic's core philosophy is based upon checking for and eliminating nervous system interference allowing brain messages to communicate clearly with the cells and body parts intended.

Bodies have been designed to experience a lifetime of wellness. Without clear messages from the brain, the cells and body parts can become misinformed or lack information. The result can be a chemical imbalance. Remember, your cells and body parts create natural body chemicals according to instructions from brain impulses.

Clear communication from the brain through the spinal cord allows the body the best opportunity for healing and sustaining optimal health.

This is why chiropractic care is leading the Wellnesscare Revolution.

Our Children's Futures

If we continue to apply "sickcare" to our infants and children, their bodies could never learn how to build wellness on their own. Children could come to believe that their bodies are just beakers full of chemicals. When their bodies show signs of breakdown, just add medication until the chemicals balance again.

As adults and parents, we are a nation of children who have now matured and are desperately hoping there is something better for our families.

We want answers beyond medication and sickcare.

We want wellness.

Wellness can be achieved at virtually any phase of life, which makes the contents of this book a life changing catalyst for anyone who is ready to begin again.

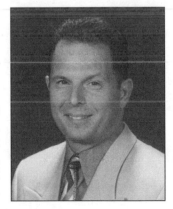

Dr. CJ Mertz
President, Chiropractic USA
and Team WLP Chiropractic
Training Organization
Austin, TX
www.teamwlp.com

PART TWO

SUBLUXATION: THE NEXT HOUSEHOLD WORD

By Dr. Greg S. Tomalin, D.C.
Dr. Amanda J. Kelley, D.C.

As chiropractors, we have always known the importance of spinal check-ups. We also understood the damage and danger caused by subluxation. What we didn't realize is how important it is that subluxation becomes a household word.

Then last year, something happened to us that changed our lives forever.

We received a call from a woman who wanted to meet for a consultation. Our office staff set an appointment for that day. When she arrived at our office, we were shocked and taken back at what we saw. Tears quickly began to fill the eyes of everyone in the waiting room, the office staff and us. Let us tell you her story.

When Theresa Sullivan was 4-years-old, she was diagnosed with epilepsy. It is a condition that, if not treated properly, can have serious consequences on your health — including death. Theresa began having uncontrollable seizures. Her medical doctor put her on Phenobarbital and other powerful drugs. Her seizures continued.

At 16, her life worsened. She began developing such severe migraines each day that she developed a sleeping disorder. She started taking more drugs. The seizures continued.

Over the next 10 years, Theresa was taking more than 10

medications. She saw more than 11 doctors and specialists. Her symptoms now included anxiety, obesity, gastro esophageal reflux disease and multiple seizures *every* single day.

Theresa became clinically depressed and lost her job. She had been told by her last doctor that she would have to live with the seizures forever. Tearfully, as a mother and wife, she knew that her children would have to continue to see their mom have seizures in front of them every day.

While thoughts of suicide entered in her mind, she knew she had to keep it together for her husband, family and God.

She decided to give one last try. Having heard about the effectiveness of chiropractic, she made her first new patient appointment. She prayed for a miracle.

It was apparent from the tired and weathered look on Theresa's face, as well as the bald patches on her head, she had been going through a war…and was losing the battle.

During her first visit, a chiropractic exam was performed which included checking her posture and taking x-rays of her spine. There was no doubt Theresa was suffering from multiple levels of subluxation in her spine. This interfered with her natural ability to regulate and heal. Theresa was told we did not treat seizures in our office. We adjust subluxation. She was ready to begin. And so were we!

What happened next was nothing short of a miracle. Within days, Theresa knew her life would never be the same.

Theresa went weeks without a single seizure. Then it was months. Almost one year later, Theresa is amazingly seizure free. Theresa noticed remarkable improvements in every aspect of her life including family and work. She lost weight and got rid of the medicines that were holding her body hostage. Through chiropractic care, she regained control of her own life! Theresa tells us that she couldn't imagine living her life without chiropractic.

This woman changed our lives forever. We now believe, more than ever, subluxation MUST become a household word. We have helped hundreds of people with hundreds of different health problems. But the truth is we have analyzed only one condition—subluxation!

So what exactly is subluxation?

It's actually pretty simple. Your brain, spinal cord and spinal nerves are responsible for controlling everything in your body. All of your muscles, organs, tissues and cells are controlled by your nervous system. Your spinal cord, which is nicknamed your "life line," is protected by 24 moveable bones, or vertebrae. In between each vertebra there is a pair of nerves branching off the spinal cord extending to different parts of your body.

A *subluxation* occurs when spinal bones, or vertebrae, become misaligned. This could cause potentially dangerous pressure on the nerves. It can also make it difficult or impossible for the nerves to function normally.

You can't really feel a subluxation. You could definitely feel the effects! These effects could be things like numbness, tingling, headaches and lower back pain. But these effects could also include more serious conditions.

If your nervous system isn't working like it should, then your body can't work like it should either!

So what causes subluxation? There are many situations in life that could cause subluxation. Things as common as car accidents, sports injuries, slip and falls, poor posture, childhood falls, gravity, the birthing process and even just life itself.

Vertebral subluxation is something you may need to manage throughout your life. It isn't something you can get rid of one time and be assured it never returns. In order to manage subluxation, first have a chiropractor check your spine for subluxation. If subluxations are found, the doctor will determine the degree and the protocol to correct them.

Then, you must regularly maintain your spine for subluxations, just as you would regularly maintain and check your teeth for cavities.

How do people know if they have subluxations? A doctor of chiropractic can properly examine and check you for subluxation. Medical doctors are rarely trained in detecting or correcting subluxations, just like chiropractors are rarely trained in performing surgery.

Subluxation is commonly referred to as the "silent killer." This is because, often times, there are no early warning signs or symptoms. The silence of subluxation is similar to diabetes or clogged arteries. Like these health conditions, subluxations can exist in your body without you knowing.

Millions of people could be walking around everyday with severe nerve interference in their bodies. Yet, they have no idea. These people could end up with health challenges.

We believe there is quite a difference between simply being "alive" and actually "living!" Chiropractors focus on keeping your nervous system functioning as optimally as possible, so you can live and enjoy life to the fullest extent!

We believe chiropractic is the fastest-growing, drugless healing profession in the world. Why? Chiropractic works! Because of the many people who have found their healing answers, subluxation is becoming a household word.

Patients thank us for "curing" them from their health problems. But, the truth is *we have never cured anyone of anything.* All we do is remove subluxation and the body *heals itself.*

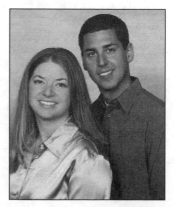

Dr. Greg S. Tomalin, D.C.
Dr. Amanda J. Kelley, D.C.
Health and Wellnes Chiropractic Center, P.C.
Broomfield, CO
720-887-0624
www.subluxationfree.com

PART THREE

CAUSE VERSUS EFFECT

By Dr. Joseph Esposito,

D.C., F.A.A.I.M., D.A.C.B.N., D.C.C.N., C.C.S.P., C.C.N., C.N.S.

One Sunday afternoon I told my son to come and eat lunch. He questioned, "Why?"

I answered, "Because it will keep you healthy."

After a silent moment he again asked, "Why?"

I answered, "Because your body needs nutrients and calories to maintain its healthy existence."

He repeated in a machine gun approach, "Why?"

What if adults did the same thing with their doctors in order to find the cause of health problems?

Your doctor says you have "migraines." You drilled with three "whys." Before your doctor can reach for the prescription pad, you might find the cause of your problem.

Many patients stop inquiring once they discover the name of their symptoms without probing further for the cause. Americans are obsessed with "diagnosis" even if it's nothing more than symptoms in Latin.

You go to your doctor with a skin rash. Your doctor sternly reports, "You have dermatitis".

You jump for joy, call your mother and rejoice, "They found the cause of my rash!"

By diagnosing you with dermatitis, your doctor merely said

the Latin version of "you have irritation and inflammation of the skin." You already knew that!

Finding the Source

By the time you experience a disease process, you may have had dysfunction for a period of time.

First, your body malfunctions. Then, you have a disease process. Lastly, you experience symptoms.

The final to arrive and the first to leave are your symptoms. The hardest to find and fix is the initial malfunction.

This is why I believe vertebral subluxations are the most overlooked health condition in the world. It is the compression or choking of one or more nerves exiting your spinal column. The nerves in your body are like wires. If the wires going to your stomach are compressed, the organ may begin to dysfunction. At this point, you may not have symptoms. Eventually, if the malfunction continues, it may produce a disease process. After the disease process continues, you eventually experience the symptom of pain.

If you are given medication to eliminate the pain and not the malfunction, you may never correct the cause of the problem. Covering up symptoms, without finding the cause, could allow the disease process to continue degrading your health.

The chiropractic profession was created to find and correct vertebral subluxations which could be the initial cause of disease processes.

Eliminating a Cough

A 38-year-old woman came to my office with a boisterous, startling cough. I was on the phone in my office with the door closed. I could hear this obnoxious cough all the way from the reception room.

My new patient was distraught, tired and in pain from coughing. She was fed up with doctors poking and prodding her to find the cause of her problem.

She said "You are my (cough) last hope (cough). I am getting (cough) married (cough) and all I want to do is say (cough) my vows without this (cough) cough."

I didn't focus on the cough or lungs but the body as a whole. I looked at her spinal column and spinal nerves. There I found a vertebral subluxation between the first and second vertebra. The misaligned vertebra was suffocating the vital nerve exiting below it.

After completing an examination and x-ray, I explained the findings. After a chiropractic adjustment and with the pressure on her nerve removed, her body was able to heal itself. Her violent coughing ended. I was invited to her wedding and witnessed her saying her vows without one single cough.

Her Story in Her Words

"I went to my family physician in November of 2000 with a terrible cough. I was diagnosed with bronchitis, prescribed an antibiotic and cough suppressant and scheduled an appointment to be seen again in ten days. With no relief, I returned to the medical doctor. I was given a chest x-ray to rule out pneumonia. The doctor said I had a bad case of bronchitis that should only last three weeks. I was prescribed a stronger antibiotic, a steroidal inhaler and prednisone cough pearls.

This continued through December, with no relief. I was coughing all day and night.

Again, I had numerous tests including: bronchoscope w/biopsy, blood test, MRI of the head and body, EMG, x-rays of the chest, bronchoesophagoscopy, barium swallow, ct scan, esophagogastroduodenoscopy and x-ray of my ribs of which I had fractured a few from the cough.

All tests came back with no problems (except for the rib fractures due to the coughing).

I was sent home after three days with a list of prescriptions including: Prednisone, Prilosec, Tessalon Pearls, Robitussin w/codeine, Motrin 600 mg., Tilade inhaler and a Nebulizer machine to be used every four hours with two different meds.

At this point I was taking eight different prescriptions and still coughing. I had seen my family physician, a heart and lung specialist, a neurologist, a gastroenterologist and an ear, nose and throat specialist.

In June, the doctor could not believe I was still coughing. He referred me to an allergist.

I was put on allergy and asthma medicine: two pills, a nose spray, an inhaler, a Nebulizer machine with two medications every four hours.

I was referred to another ear, nose, & throat specialist. He prescribed more medications and an appointment to discuss sinus surgery. I was getting married and decided to schedule the procedure after my honeymoon.

On October 1, I had an appointment with Dr. Joe Esposito. My sister referred me. I was given an exam, x-rays and told to return on October 3. On October 3, just ten days before my wedding day, I was given an adjustment for a subluxation in my neck and scheduled to be seen two days later.

I returned to Dr. Esposito on October 5 with no cough at all. I felt like a new person.

On October 13, I had a beautiful wedding. I said my vows without a cough. Dr. Joe Esposito was there along with my family and friends who thanked him for giving me this miracle. For the first time in eleven months, I was without a cough.

Although my medical bills and prescriptions totaled nearly $20,000, I was most upset by all the medications which went through my body needlessly, the length of time I was on medications and the unnecessary surgical procedure the doctor wanted to do on my sinuses."

Neck Pain and More

Another patient was a young girl with mild neck pain. I asked for any other health concerns. She had been vomiting many times a day since she was five years old.

I found a subluxation in her middle back disallowing her body to function normally. I began to remove the nerve compression with repetitive spinal adjustments two to three times a week.

Her mother shares the story:

"Ten years ago, at the age of 5, my daughter began vomiting. A test done by our local pediatrician indicated the problem was an irritated epiglottis that would go away on its own.

After two weeks of no improvement, I insisted she by referred to a specialist. By this time she was vomiting, small amounts, more that a hundred times a day. It had become a constant thing.

The next doctor did testing and suggested surgery that would make it impossible for her to vomit. Although this would eliminate the immediate problem of vomiting, it did not deal with the cause.

This surgery would have also created a lifelong situation where she would be in the emergency room getting her stomach pumped every time she was sick or ate something that didn't agree with her and vomiting was necessary.

We refused the surgery. The doctor prescribed Reglan, which reduced vomiting frequency. The doctor assured me there were no adverse side effects. I later discovered long term use could cause permanent neurological problems.

I immediately took her off the drug and made an appointment for her at a very well-known hospital. She was examined by the head of pediatric gastroenterology and a gastroenterology doctor. The diagnosis was rumination, a reflexive habit of vomiting. It was their belief amoxicillin, which she was taking at the time this started, irritated her stomach causing vomiting. By continuing to take it, she vomited enough that it became a reflexive habit of her stomach.

While all of this was going on, my daughter also had a habit of cracking her back. A co-worker of mine was seeing Dr. Esposito. At my daughter's first exam, he discovered a subluxation of the spine where nerves control digestion.

Dr. Esposito recommended a chiropractic care plan. Although I must admit, I was more than a little skeptical. After 10 years of doctors, it was hard to believe a chiropractor would solve the problem.

Dr. Esposito said we could expect to begin seeing some change in about 3 months. I was surprised when, after only 3 weeks, my daughter hadn't vomited at all that day. Although we should have been jumping for joy, we were both afraid to get our hopes too high.

When the next day came and went with no vomiting, we began to get excited. Not once in the almost 10 years had she gone two days in a row without vomiting. Two days became three months. The vomiting is gone."

This sweet young girl came to my office to thank me. I waited until she left and tears ran down my face. It confirmed why I do what I do.

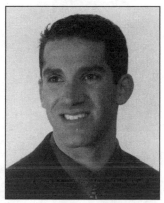

Dr. Joseph Esposito,
D.C., F.A.A.I.M., D.A.C.B.N., D.C.C.N.,
C.C.S.P., C.C.N., C.N.S.
Health Solutions
Bloomington, IL
309-665-0777
www.healthsolutions.net
Esposito@healthsolutions.net

In addition to being a doctor of chiropractic, Dr. Joseph Esposito is a Fellow of the American Association of Integrative Medicine, a board certified Naturopathic Physician, Diplomat of the American Chiropractic Board of Nutrition, Diplomat of the Gonstead System of Chiropractic, Diplomat of the College of Clinical Nutrition, Certified Chiropractic Sports Physician, Certified Clinical Nutritionist and Certified Nutrition Specialist. Dr. Joseph also has clinics in Morton, IL and Woodstock, GA.

PART FOUR

Making Subluxation a Household Word

❧

By Dr. Sandra R.H. Childers, D.C. and
Dr. Kirk Childers, D.C.

"Sub...lux...what?!", patients often ask us when we explain to them the findings of their initial evaluation. "Subluxation," we reply. "It's pronounced *sub-luks-ay-shun*."

"What is it? How did I get it? How do I get rid of it? How do I keep it from affecting my health? Or my family's health?"

In our practice, we hear questions like these every day. The key to understanding the benefits of chiropractic care lies in understanding basic principles beginning with one word: subluxation.

What is Subluxation?

Chiropractic care revolves around a process called "subluxation," which is a misalignment of the bones of the spine. These misalignments produce serious pressure on the nerve roots of the spine, which could disconnect the brain's ability to communicate with the rest of the body.

Listen to a car radio when signals become distorted by mountains or other obstructions blocking out communication from the radio station. Subluxations can be like the mountain in the way of the radio wave. These spinal misalignments could obstruct brain communication from reaching the rest of the body.

The result of this interference between brain and body manifests itself in different ways.

Often, people are not aware of the presence of subluxations. We call subluxations "silent killers" which don't always present obvious symptoms. Only a small fraction of the nerves in your body can even perceive pain. Therefore, just because you feel fine does not always mean the function of your nervous system is working at an optimal level.

When left undetected, subluxations could develop into any disease process. Disease may manifest as symptoms or "body signals." These signals may surface as numbness or tingling in the limbs, acid reflux or indigestion to a general feeling of listlessness or malaise, even constipation and diarrhea. Other signals range from back or neck pain to headaches or arm pain.

Pain is not the only red flag for subluxation. Pain is *not* what should determine your health.

Hundreds of common ailments could be directly attributed to subluxation, such as sinus problems, allergies and sleep disorders.

Every tissue and organ in the body communicates with the brain through nerves running through the spinal column. If the condition of the spine and nervous system is compromised, so could be the body's balance of health and well-being.

What Causes Subluxation?

In the simplest terms, the cause of subluxations could be narrowed down to stress in three main categories: physical, chemical and emotional.

Physical Stress

Stress which is greater than the body's internal resistance could cause subluxations. When the body experiences physical trauma, like an injury, or when the body's muscle tissue, ligaments or tendons change and react to such stressors, the spine could be affected.

Slips and falls, auto accidents, sports-related injuries or similar trauma are a few of the more obvious physical stressors. People most often associate these with the need for chiropractic care. Poor exercise habits, incorrect posture and even the birth process itself could also produce subluxations.

Chemical Stress

Chemical stress occurs when body chemistry changes as a result of overeating or consuming too much sugar, salt or fat. Chemical stress could also come from absorbing pesticides or environmental pollutants which may be present in the food we eat. Poor nutrition could result in chemical imbalances.

Body chemistry affects muscle tone. If the muscles cannot correctly support the body, the spine could suffer undue stress. Ultimately subluxations could occur.

Emotional Stress

Mental or emotional stressors, created by the demands of life, are something we all experience to one extent or another. Managing relationships with family and friends, meeting deadlines at work, fighting traffic or balancing the checkbook all contribute to our stress levels. Tension, fear, anxiety and worry often manifest themselves physically as tight muscles and ligaments, which could cause subluxation.

Every day, the nervous system is bombarded with numerous challenges. The cumulative effects of physical, chemical and emotional stress could result in tissue damage. This could take a toll on the nervous system and normal body functioning. With such a high volume of stressors in our lives, we believe everyone should be checked regularly for spinal misalignments.

How are Subluxations Detected and Managed?

Licensed Doctors of Chiropractic are specially trained to detect and manage subluxations. By undergoing a thorough evaluation, (which includes a posture check; palpation, or feeling of the spine with the hands; x-rays of the spine and possibly a computerized spinal EMG and thermography) a chiropractor can determine if you have spinal misalignments. Your chiropractor can also establish how serious they are, how many you may have and how long they have been present.

Then, by performing very precise procedures called spinal adjustments, the chiropractor can begin to restore the spine to its proper position. Adjustments over time could remove the life-choking stress placed on the nervous system.

By correcting and maintaining proper alignment of the spine through regular adjustments, a wellness chiropractor can help patients achieve optimal health. This could include pain relief and increased range of motion in muscles and joints. It could even include improved blood circulation, blood pressure reduction and increased endorphin levels.

There are a number of techniques used by chiropractors to adjust subluxation. Those techniques differ according to the type of stress affecting the spine.

"Why Hasn't My Medical Doctor Told Me About Subluxation?"

We took the time to actually ask many of our friends in the medical field this very question. These doctors held degrees in a variety of medical specialties including pediatrics, general medicine, neurosurgery and pathology.

What we learned is there are many explanations as to why medical doctors fail to recognize or address subluxation. Here are the answers they gave most often:

- Medical doctors are simply not trained to detect the presence of subluxations of the spine and are, therefore, not aware of the effects or benefits of wellness chiropractic care.

- Some thought chiropractic care was only good for lower back pain.

- They subscribe to a different school of thought as to what constitutes the concept of health. Medical college curriculums focus on traditional or mainstream medicine designed to treat existing disease, illness and injury.

It's an age-old battle of sickcare versus wellnesscare and prevention. Over 25 million chiropractic patients have already made, what we view as, the right choice.

Doctors of chiropractic are trained to look for the *causes* of diseases, illnesses and injuries as they relate to the spine and nervous system. Once detected, chiropractors apply techniques for the body to correct and treat its own infirmities with the goal of preventing future health problems.

Some medical doctors are uninformed about the process of subluxation and the benefits of chiropractic care. As a result, they may not recognize chiropractic care as a "valid" means of health care and maintenance.

Unfortunately, in doing so, they deny their patients the opportunity to benefit from this highly specialized and proven form of health care.

An abundance of information about chiropractic care is available from many sources, including the Internet and legitimate professional organizations like:

International Chiropractors Association
(www.chiropractic.org)

International Chiropractic Pediatric Association
(www.icpa4kids.org)

Journal of Vertebral Subluxation Research
(www.jsvr.com)

Today, as the public awareness of health care options grows and the demands for alternatives to drug-based and surgical remedies increase, more and more people are exploring the benefits and solutions offered by chiropractic care.

More Than Just Back Pain?

Absolutely!

We're not just back and neck pain doctors. By detecting and correcting subluxation, we can help improve any number of common health complaints and discomforts. By maintaining the spine and nervous system, we can help prevent many health problems before they occur.

Patients come to us after visiting other medical professionals with little or no results. We imagine the frustration (and expense!) which could have been avoided if they had visited a chiropractor first.

Keith experienced back pain for twenty years. He visited many doctors and physical therapy with no success. Keith told us, "For the first time ever, a doctor was able to identify the source of my pains…subluxation. Not only has my back felt better, my overall health has improved to the point where I am enjoying things I haven't been able to do for years."

Still, chiropractic care is often sought as a "last resort." Subluxation and spinal misalignment can affect general health and well-being. Understanding this can help us make better decisions about how we care for our bodies and maintain good health.

One family learned the devastating effects of subluxations when they brought in their 9-month-old son for a spinal checkup. Jacob was a very sick little boy. He had been suffering from ear infections since he was born. It had been several weeks since Jacob or his parents had slept a full night.

Jacob's eyes were red and watery with thick mucous running from his ears, nose and mouth. He had been prescribed several rounds of antibiotics and tubes for his ears with no resolution of his condition.

We examined Jacob and found he had subluxations. We began adjusting his spine to help restore his body's own health potential.

Today, Jacob is four years old and continues to receive spinal maintenance. He has not suffered from inner ear infections since!

Chiropractic care is a drug-free, surgical-free and preventive measure that can be performed on all patients, regardless of age or physical condition.

Knowing what subluxation is and the potentially devastating effects on you and your body, wouldn't you agree it's time to have your spine checked by a Doctor of Chiropractic?

Your body has an innate ability to heal and protect itself. The sooner you get checked, the sooner you could be on the road to optimal health.

Now you have learned the meaning of "subluxation." Don't keep it to yourself! You can educate and inform others.

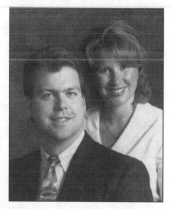

Dr. Sandra R.H. Childers, D.C.
Dr. Kirk Childers, D.C.
University Chiropractic
Durham, NC
919-493-1940
www.chiropracticforlife.com

PART FIVE

Chiropractic Care for a Healthy Lifestyle

❦

By Dr. Randall B. Johns, D.C.

At 5:00 a.m. after hitting the snooze button for the third time, he crawled out of bed and made an important decision. This was the same decision he made for the past seven years at least five days a week…a morning jog. The jog had become a staple in his daily routine.

At age 37, he realized he was not getting any younger. So he incorporated exercise into his daily rituals. He felt perfectly healthy. In fact, John really had no health concerns at all.

He had a wonderful marriage of nine years and two beautiful children and a great career with a stable company. John exercised a minimum of five days a week, drank plenty of clean, purified water, and weighed within 10 pounds of his 175-pound frame from high school days.

This year, like all the others, John had been given a clean bill of health from his doctor. Without a doubt, he felt great and did all the right things to maintain a healthy lifestyle…or did he?

After a 10-minute stretch, John began his morning ritual. After running a few minutes, the rhythmic sound of his feet hitting the hard ground beneath him had become peaceful. He pictured eating breakfast and reading the morning paper before heading to work. He found happiness in thoughts of cuddling with his wife for a brief moment before they lovingly woke their two children for school.

Unfortunately, John never made it back home. Suffering from a massive heart attack, his precious life was dramatically cut short of his God-given potential.

Heart disease did not run in his family. He did everything his doctors advised and had complete trust in the healthcare system. How could such a man die suddenly from a heart attack?

While John is a fictional character, his story resembles real life tragedy. Every day in America, people die of heart attacks without prior warning.

Interestingly, in a large percentage of people suffering a heart attack, the first symptom is not chest pain, but sudden death! People who base health on how they feel, could be playing a deadly game of Russian roulette. John, like millions of other people in the world, never took time to be checked for vertebral subluxation.

My name is Dr. Randall Johns and I want to provide you with valuable information that which could forever change the way you and your family think about health. First, let me share a little about myself.

I am a doctor of chiropractic with an office in Texarkana, located in the northeast corner of Texas. This is where I was born, raised and still live. My staff and I serve hundreds of patients weekly, which include checking for vertebral subluxation.

What is Subluxation?

Subluxation is a shift in the spine causing interference to the nervous system. As a chiropractor specializing in the correction of vertebral subluxation, I am very passionate and excited about what I do. Each day, I have the opportunity to help people reach their optimal potential to express 100% life force. God created an amazing body and inside of each person placed the gift of healing. This God-given healing happens from inside your body to the outside.

The innate wisdom inside each person is evident in all living creatures. Subluxations interfere with innate wisdom and could cause sickness and disease.

Think of it this way, what happens when a person cuts his or her finger? The body begins to bleed at the site of the wound. This eventually clots and forms a scab. Within approximately two weeks, the cut is healed.

Most people have never thought of themselves as being healers. But, that is exactly what they are because God created them that way.

Automatically You

When a person walks into a very cold room, the body begins to shake and shiver generating energy to stay warm. In contrast, when a person walks into a stifling hot room, the body begins to sweat as a means of staying cool.

What makes this so amazing is the body acts on autopilot without any thought or direction from the person. The body knows automatically, 24-hours a day, how to heal and regulate all functions.

What inside your body is automatically controlling and co-ordinating your functions? It is your nervous system, which is comprised of your brain and spinal cord.

Your innate wisdom is expressed through your brain and spinal cord, which is highly protected by 24 moveable bones known as vertebrae. The nervous system, which is the lifeline to the body, is the only organ in the body encased by bone.

Subluxations or misalignments of the spinal bones interfere with the vital communication from the brain up-and-down the spinal cord to the body.

All 100 trillion cells are directly controlled by this complex and intricate system. A person's heart is supposed to beat more than 100,000 times each day. If a subluxation is affecting the nerve going to the heart, I want it removed so I get all 100,000 beats!

I view chiropractic, not as a treatment but as a lifestyle to be healthy. It is a life principle that revolves around a healthy, functioning spine and nervous system.

As a chiropractor, I have patients come to me with various health challenges. Rather than provide patients with yet another treatment to handle their symptoms, I check for interferences caused by subluxation to the nervous system. Then, I correct the problem. The body takes care of the healing.

I am concerned about the well-being of children and adults. Unfortunately, we live in a society believing our bodies heal from outside in. Let's take a look at how some deal with health.

Upon giving birth, women receive epidurals; both the mother and the unborn child are medicated. As the child grows, he or she is immunized and given cough syrup, cold medicine, baby aspirin and other types of drugs. By the time the child reaches early school years, he or she is put on behavioral medication. When the child reaches teenage years, he or she starts taking appetite suppressants and psychotropic drugs for depression or anxiety.

With such a system, how can children take parents seriously when told to "just say no to drugs?"

Could it be children are being conditioned their entire lives that pain, sickness and behavior are drug deficiencies?

According to *Health Affairs*, March/April 2002; 21; 207-217, government actuaries report U.S. healthcare spending will top $2.8 *trillion* by 2011.

This means by 2011 the annual American healthcare spending will rise to $9,216 *per person* which is double the amount in 2000.

Do you look forward to spending over $9,000 a year on fighting illness?

Why with nearly 1.5 trillion dollars spent on healthcare in

America in 2000, does America rank 37th in *The World Health Organization's Ranking of the World's Health Systems?*

It is easy to see that our healthcare system and beliefs are, in my opinion, in need of help. Could this be a "sick care" system focusing on treating sickness and disease through medication and surgery, rather than a wellness system focused on preventing sickness and disease in the first place? Could it be some have forgotten where true healing comes from?

In my opinion, doctors are not the ones who heal anything. It's the body that heals itself!

Please understand having a medical system in place is important. I believe the new model of healthcare will revolve around a philosophy of healing coming from above-down and inside-out.

Everything in life is made possible in direct correlation to a person's level of health. Every single person deserves to be checked for subluxation at least once in life, possibly being the most important health decision ever made.

All we can ask for in life is to have the best possible chance to be healthy and well. My goal is to educate people and give them the opportunity of health and wellness. I would encourage you and your loved ones to be checked for subluxation so life can be enjoyed to the fullest.

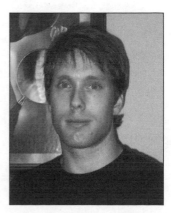

Dr. Randall "Randy" B. Johns, D.C.
Johns Family Chiropractic
Texarkana, TX
903-223-8776

PART SIX

WELLNESS...
THE NEXT FRONTIER

By Dr. Steve Waddell, D.C.

Who among us doesn't want to live a longer, better life?

Over the decades, our quest for longevity and vitality has, at times, been a somewhat frustrating and confusing chase. Social and "pseudo-scientific" trends have attempted to dictate the choices we've made about how we take care of our bodies. Some of those choices were good, others disastrous. At best, we've managed to maintain a certain level of healthiness and well-being. At worst, we've surrendered the responsibilities of our own health.

Today, as the cost of health care continues to rise, we've come to a noticeable crossroad in our quest. Do we stumble blindly along the well-worn path of conformity, which, by the way, could be becoming increasingly convoluted? Or do we arm ourselves with information and blaze a trail of our own toward optimum health?

For many people, the answer is clear. They've experienced a growing sense of disillusionment and disappointment with a system which could be tainted by politics and big business. This sense of betrayal has sparked within them the desire and determination to reclaim responsibility for their own well-being.

Much of the stimulus behind this movement is fueled by the

desire of baby boomers to live longer and better, their willingness to take personal responsibility for their own health and, if necessary, spend money out of their own pockets. These folks are typically willing to ask hard questions and unwilling to settle for pat answers. They are willing to question the wisdom of simply handing their bodies, minds and spirits over to any institution, government or insurance company.

In doing so, they've sought other, less traditional approaches to health care. From this, the buzzword "alternative health care" was born.

No Alternative to Alternative Health Care

In *Journal of the American Medical Association (JAMA)*, November 11, 1998, a report by Dr. David M. Eisenberg, MD revealed, "Extrapolations to the US population suggest a 47.3% increase in total visits to alternative medicine practitioners from 427 million in 1990 to 629 million in 1997, **thereby exceeding total visits to all US primary care physicians.** Estimated expenditures for alternative medicine professional services increased 45.2% between 1990 and 1997 and were conservatively estimated at $21.2 billion in 1997 with at least $12.2 billion paid out-of-pocket."

The trend continues to grow. It can now be argued "mainstream" medicine is quickly becoming "alternative" and that "alternative" health care is now mainstream.

The current use of the term "alternative" implies you have a choice.

It's also imperative you explore "No Alternative" health care — those things you must do to keep your body and its systems performing at peak levels. You cannot ignore what your body requires if you are seeking to achieve and maintain optimal health. A colleague of mine, Dr. Mark Percival of Ontario, coined the phrase. He stated health education remains the missing link in our health care system.

Education, not medicine, is the very foundation of health care. When health education is inadequate, people become increasingly reliant upon medical intervention expecting miracles. Percival's theory of "No Alternative" health care encourages people to stop for a moment and consider: What are the benefits derived from "no alternative" behaviors such as subluxation-free nerve systems, nutritious eating, rest, exercise, recreation, self-reflection, caring relationships, creative expression and fulfilling vocations?

All are essential to health. In my opinion, there are no alternatives to them. No pill or therapy can remove the ill effects caused by stress, injury, poor posture, junk food, lack of exercise and recreation, insufficient rest, worry, fear, resentment, ignorance, poor relationships and unsatisfying, distressing or even unhealthy work.

Wellness or Crisis? Which Do You Prefer?

Traditionally, medical physicians treat existing diseases and provide emergency crisis care. On a recent airplane flight, I sat next to a cancer doctor from a very prestigious clinic. In talking about our careers, she made a vital observation.

"Dr. Waddell, you know, nothing I do even closely resembles 'health' care. You can't call it health care and you certainly can't call it wellness," she said. "It's disease care."

In my experience, doctors of chiropractic provide health care and lead their patients toward wellness.

Wellness Everywhere

Wellness, it seems, is everywhere you look. Wellness means something different to everyone you ask. Thousands of products and services are marketed and advertised under the wellness umbrella. Many industries — food, fitness, drugs, diets, electronics, cosmetics and so on — have claimed their share of the market.

Ask someone to define wellness. They might say it's having six-pack abs...wrinkle-free skin...eating organic food...taking this supplement or that vitamin...using this skin cream...buying that gadget.

I believe true wellness is a condition. It is not a commodity. It cannot be bought or sold. It cannot be artificially produced or synthetically duplicated. It must be achieved through means familiar to most baby boomers: education, determination and plain, old hard work.

In this age of unprecedented prosperity, when we have access to conveniences our grandparents never dreamed of, the notions of hard work and perseverance have taken on negative connotations. But when it comes to achieving and maintaining optimal health, there is still no better substitute.

Wellness Formulas to Live By

Most every physiologist on the planet knows, second-by-second, your body is breaking down. They also know, second-by-second, your body is rebuilding.

My colleague, mentor and friend, Dr. C.J. Mertz, puts it this way, "When the breaking down process (B), exceeds the rebuilding process (R), your body is in a state of 'dis-ease' (a lack of ease). Your body is not performing as it should. This invariably leads to disease."

The first formula: B>R = DIS-EASE = DISEASE

He continues, "When the rebuilding process (R), exceeds the breaking down (B), your body is in a state of wellness and performing at its optimum. Health and healing are yours."

The second formula: R>B = WELLNESS

The Key to Wellness...A Healthy Nervous System

The rebuilding process is under the control of and dependent upon nerve supply. To achieve wellness, you must insure the nervous system is fully empowered to perform the automatic, routine maintenance necessary to support the rebuilding process.

I feel the best way to do this is to have your spine and nerve system checked for subluxation. A wellness chiropractic checkup focuses on the relationship between your spine's structure and the function of the nervous system.

Imagine this. Suppose you have a chair with one leg shorter or weaker than the others. Would you agree its structure is off? It looks like a chair, but it doesn't work like a chair.

Your body works the same way. If your structure is off due to subluxation (misalignment of the vertebrae, poor posture or loss of normal spinal curves), then your nerve supply could be compromised and your body doesn't work correctly.

Information, Application, Dedication

When it comes to the state of your health and well being, take a cue from the baby boomer generation and don't settle for pat answers or quick fixes. Get information from reliable sources, including licensed doctors of chiropractic.

Now that you know what wellness is and how to achieve and maintain it, turn that knowledge into wisdom by applying it. Make an honest assessment of your current level of wellness. With the help of your chiropractor — your wellness expert — map out a plan for achieving optimal health and healing by using all the health care resources available to you.

Dedication and determination will be your best governing tools in the quest for optimal health and healing. A steadfast commitment to take responsibility for your own health will make you an active participant in discovering wellness...the next frontier.

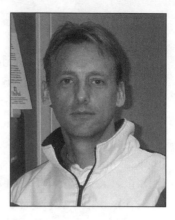

Dr. Steve Waddell, D.C.
Wellness Coach™ Chiropractic
Red Deer, Alberta, Canada
403-342-7670
drwaddell.wellnesscoach@shaw.ca

Dr. Steve Waddell, D.C., is President and Head Coach of Wellness Coach™. An internationally recognized wellness expert, author, publisher, lecturer and practicing chiropractor, Dr. Waddell can be reached at drwaddell.wellnesscoach@shaw.ca

PART SEVEN

CHIROPRACTIC WELLNESS = PROACTIVE HEALTH CARE

❦

By Dr. Robert Vasquez, D.C.

The choices we make could be much more important to our wellness than we realize. Knowledge of what is happening inside our bodies helps us understand the changes we could make outside, which could lead to happier, healthier lives.

Many health problems could be alleviated before they start by assuring the body's nervous system is functioning optimally. The spine, which houses our nervous system, needs to be properly aligned so nerve signals can freely flow to each part of our bodies.

I know this is true from personal experience. My first encounter with chiropractic was nothing short of miraculous.

From childhood well into my adult years, I suffered headaches every day. I couldn't remember a time when I didn't have them. My career goal was to become a medical doctor. While taking pre-med courses in college, I asked instructors what was causing my headaches. They could never tell me the cause; but they did recommend I take lots of different medications to treat the pain.

That approach didn't make sense to me because I knew God didn't create junk. The headaches had to be caused by something other than not having enough medication in my body.

At the same time, my sister began seeing improvements in

her allergies, sinuses and headaches during chiropractic care. Encouraged, I went to her chiropractor to see if I could get relief from my headaches and find out what chiropractic was all about.

The doctor told me my spine had a condition called subluxation, a type of misalignment that was placing pressure on my nervous system and causing my headaches. I was excited because I felt someone could finally give me a cause for my condition instead of just treating the symptoms.

After receiving a series of chiropractic adjustments, I realized I had been pain-free for a month without medication. Before the adjustments, I had taken three over-the-counter pain relievers every morning and every night, as long as I could remember, so I could be headache-free.

I was so amazed by this transformation, and what this doctor was able to do for me, I wanted to share my results with others. I left the pre-med program and began chiropractic college studying for my chiropractic doctorate.

An Apple a Day. An Adjustment a Week.

Weekly spinal adjustments are as much a part of my life as brushing my teeth. As a doctor of chiropractic, I have weekly adjustments to maintain the health of my spine and nervous system. This allows my body to function optimally and give it the best chance to naturally fight off any health problems.

I consider chiropractic wellness as proactive health care. We all understand the importance of maintaining our automobiles to keep them running smoothly. We don't wait until our engine seizes up before we have an oil change. Usually a person checks and adds oil before low oil becomes a costly reality.

Why not take care of your spine and nervous system before the body seizes up? After all, the nervous system controls all functions taking place in your body.

Most people experience what I call "reactive health care."

After getting sick and going to the doctor one might receive medication to treat the symptoms, which in turn could cover up the cause of the illness. The condition could continue. But we may not be aware of it because we no longer have symptoms. As a result, our bodies may no longer be functioning at their best.

What can be done to keep our bodies in good working order? I believe keeping our nervous systems healthy can make a huge difference. In my office, I generally see three causes of spinal subluxation:

- Chemical stress. Obvious things like the use of alcohol and cigarettes can affect our nervous system. Less obvious things could also affect the nervous system, such as prescription and over-the-counter medication. Additives in food, including sugar, can also affect our health. We have a lot of control over what we put in our mouths and ultimately our bodies. My rule of thumb is if you can't pronounce it, you shouldn't eat it!

- Physical stress. Subluxation could occur as a result of poor posture, falls, slips, vehicle accidents, poor sleeping habits, sports or sitting improperly. Only a tiny fraction of the nervous system feels pain, so many people may not realize their spines are subluxated. By the time pain is present, the patient could have suffered subluxation for weeks, months or even years, possibly causing irreversible damage.

- Emotional stress. At times, life may be difficult. Stress, tension, anxiety and depression can cause muscle tension that could affect the spine.

A common phrase is, "stress kills." Stress has a significant impact on your entire body, particularly, the health of the nervous system.

I see subluxations caused by emotional issues most often among my patients. This is why I encourage patients to change their outlooks on life. We recommend attending workshops on stress reduction, goal setting and other issues to help patients better cope with their fast-paced lives. Sometimes a patient may choose to end an unhealthy relationship or a high-stress job. This could remove the muscular tension which could be causing the subluxation.

Subluxation can happen the moment we enter the world! The perfect spine of a fetus could be subluxated through the process of birth. This could be just the beginning.

Babies begin to crawl and sit up. Sometimes parents put them in walkers. The baby may not be prepared to stand yet. The forces of gravity may place unwanted stress on tiny spines causing subluxation.

Then, the baby begins to walk. As any parent knows, learning to walk means frequent falls. Every time the baby falls, more stress is placed on the spine. Again, subluxation could result.

The baby becomes a child who is sometimes sick with childhood colds and infections. Parents, wanting the best for their child, may give medications like cough suppressants. Inadvertently, by giving the child medicines, the parents could cause chemical subluxation.

By first grade, the child's teacher is concerned. The child may not be able to sit still and is showing behaviorial issues. The teacher wants testing for Attention Deficit Disorder. The child receives a prescription medication to aid concentration during the day and one to help him or her sleep at night. These powerful drugs could cause side effects which could harm the health of the nervous system.

Then there is sports, a vehicle accident as a teen-ager or a high-stress job as an adult.

The healthy baby who once had a perfectly functioning spine and nervous system could now be a mess! Sometimes, by this point, the spine may or may not be able to be restored to its original state. However, chiropractic care can offer a person a better quality of life.

It's easy for me to see subluxation when I look at a patient's posture. I see posture as an outward expression of what is going on inside the body. One shoulder may be higher than the other, the spine is not straight from a back view or the head is tilted to one side. These are signs the patient's nervous system could be kinked, pinched or stretched.

What most people don't understand about the nervous system is that we *cannot* survive without it. The nervous system controls every function of the body, therefore subluxations, directly or indirectly, could produce thousands of effects which could shut off life.

Here are some of the success stories I've seen in my office after patients with subluxations decide to receive care and modify their lifestyle choices:

- A mother-to-be had an overall feeling of wellness during her pregnancy – no back or pelvic pain, no swelling or feelings of discomfort. She said she couldn't imagine going through her pregnancy without chiropractic.

- An autistic boy began to have emotions at appropriate times.

- A pre-schooler's chronic ear infections disappeared.

- A stressed-out mom became relaxed, happy and pain-free.

- A patient with migraine headaches is free of pain, and said she no longer feels like a bird trapped in a cage.

These are just a few of our success stories. But I've found people can benefit from having a healthy functioning spine and nervous system. My passion is to educate and teach people to have their families checked for subluxations. By removing subluxations, people could expect to live healthier lives. My dream is to have patients, and their whole families, undergoing proactive care.

The Roman poet and satirist Juvenal said, "A sound mind in a sound body is a thing to be prayed for."

I say, "A sound mind and a sound body is a thing to be adjusted for."

Both are imperative to maintaining wellness.

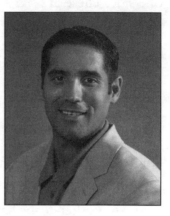

Dr. Robert Vasquez, D.C.
Vasquez Family Chiropractic
Bedford, TX
(817) 267-0102

PART EIGHT

SPINAL MAINTENANCE

❧

By Dr. Howard I. Werfel, D.C.

In the past 100 years, science has made technological advances that have improved the human condition and the ability of people to lead longer and healthier lives.

I believe the advancements we have made, however, pale in comparison to the understanding discovered over a hundred years ago that our bodies are self regulating, self developing and self healing entities.

Chiropractic was born in Davenport, Iowa in 1895 when D.D. Palmer realized a vertebra could lose its normal position and cause interference between the brain and the body. By applying a specific corrective force, called a chiropractic adjustment, the nerve interference could be removed and the normal function of the body restored.

In my experience, there has never been a profession more capable to unleash the true healing powers of the human body as chiropractic.

The nervous system controls and coordinates the body's cells, tissues, organs and systems. Disease could be caused if the body experiences functional interference or loss of control. Infectious diseases are the loss of the immune system's ability to function normally. Restore immune system function and the infection could be handled by the body's normal healing responses.

Whenever you see a miracle of healing or a spontaneous remission of "terminal" illness, you are witnessing internal intelligence regaining its incredible ability to recreate.

One of the beliefs of chiropractic, which I subscribe to wholeheartedly, is if the nerve system is returned to its optimum state of function, then whatever diseases an individual may have would resolve with no need to treat the specific disease.

Simply said, I believe, the future of health care will be focused on correcting the cause of diseases through chiropractic care. Included in this will be spinal adjustments, nutritional improvement, exercise and mental or emotional conditioning.

It seems, at times, answers are more obvious and simple than most of us are willing to see. We are capable of a higher level of health and wellness than many believe. It is time we start questioning.

What is responsible for our creation from one cell into a multi-billion cell organism?

What is responsible for converting the food we eat into power to recreate our bodies cell-by-cell, second-by-second, every day of our lives?

Spinal Maintenance: A Whole New Level of Health

Chiropractic doctors look for and treat causes, not merely symptoms. I believe if the cause of nervous system interference is corrected, the body will heal with no attention to the disease itself.

If a nerve died in one of your teeth, the tooth itself would die shortly after. The same is true of interference with a nerve responsible for the health of one of your vital organs. Cut the nerve to the organ and the organ could begin to produce disease and die.

A majority of our culture has been trained to treat disease, first, with drugs. People have been conditioned to believe heart disease, strokes and cancers are "normal" results of aging in the human body.

I don't view disease as a normal function of aging. Rather, I see it as an outcome of a body not maintained, and a nerve system not in healthy, working order.

Health is not exclusively about how you feel. Your health is in your control. Don't wait for signs of breakdown and plan to treat the crisis with drugs and surgery. This is not wellness. I believe it violates the basic laws of life and disrespects the body's inborn, innate healing ability.

This inborn healing ability flows from the brain, through the spinal cord and out through the nerves to all body parts. We were meant to be well. The proof is in the results chiropractors continue to produce.

Dr. Howard I. Werfel, D.C.
Werfel Chiropractic Center
Suffern, NY
845-368-4100

PART NINE

A LIMITLESS POSSIBILITY TO HEALING

❧

By Dr. Gregory J. Sabatino, D.C.

How can we put limitations on the limitless? How can we bind the boundless? When we truly understand the source of all healing, we can better understand its unlimited potential.

I believe the power that created life is the same power and infinite wisdom which created the universe. This power exists as inner wisdom within the body and its healing potential is limitless.

As doctors, we may place physical limitations on the body's ability to heal. In turn, we limit ourselves as healers.

When we diagnose a disease or illness by giving it an exact name we claim the disease into reality. We then set restrictions on healing by giving a prognosis. With a prognosis we could actually be imprisoning the patient in a kind of "life sentence."

"Your prognosis is terminal. You only have two weeks to live."

While we may close possibilities with a prognosis, we need to open the possibilities of healing. I believe we have a limitless possibility to heal. I chose to never close any healing possibility by naming a certain disease or illness.

In chiropractic, we know all disease is simply a dis-ease. A lack of ease in the body just waiting to return to the harmonious ease of its natural state. Through a dynamic healing force in the human spine, I free the body's inner wisdom for limitless possibilities of healing.

I believe miracles happen. During my 13 years as a chiropractor, I have come from a point of non-belief to a place of limitless possibility.

I graduated December 1990 from Los Angeles College of Chiropractic. I had confidence and belief in medicine and therapy machines, more so than I did in the ability of my two hands to manifest healing in the human body through chiropractic care.

The more healing I witnessed through my patients, the stronger my belief became in chiropractic and myself. I have humbled myself to the realization I am a mere vehicle through which, I believe, God has manifested healing for myself and my patients.

I believe when limitless healing possibilities became my reality, true miracles began to manifest in my practice. My belief has become a certainty of chiropractic and an expectation of healing.

Healing Manifested

At the time, Sandra suffered from multiple medical conditions including fibromyalgia and severe asthma. She was taking 17 different medications daily including four asthma inhalers of varying strengths. After her first chiropractic adjustment she began to cry tears of joy.

Unable to breathe deeply the evening before her first chiropractic appointment, Sandra had spent the entire night in the hospital hooked up to a breathing machine having powerful asthma medications pumped into her lungs.

After only two very specific chiropractic adjustments to her spine, she was able to breathe deeper and clearer than she had in her entire life. Over the next two months, she reduced her daily intake of medications from 17 to only one per day.

Olga came with multiple sclerosis. Diagnosed by MRI studies, Olga had characteristic symptoms to match. She had visual disturbances, sensitivity to light, electric shock sensations and uncontrolled motor function. She had been given twelve different prescriptions to take over the past two years without noticeable results but with painful side effects.

I aligned her spine to allow the inner wisdom of her body to begin the healing process. For Olga's first adjustment, I realigned the top two bones in her neck, the atlas and axis.

Her vision became normal, her balance greatly improved and she was able to walk straight without any noticeable deficit. She was told by her doctors she is now in remission. Could remission be the body healing itself?

Olga has truly been a blessing showing me the power of faith and belief. Olga has told me she believes God sent her to me. She said if it wasn't for me and my office, she would have given up on life and hope.

Through my experiences with Olga and many patients like her, I realize it is not just chiropractic that does the healing. Love, hope and belief also heal.

I believe healing through chiropractic could happen without the patient believing. Five years prior to his first visit at my office, Leroy had suffered multiple strokes. He was left with severe and constant headaches, dizziness and loss of balance. One side of his face had no sensation.

Within the first week of my care, his headaches, dizziness, loss of balance and facial numbness were 99.9 % gone.

During the following visit, Leroy had a confession, "Doc, when you first told me you could help me, I didn't believe you. I have been suffering for over five years and had been under the care of many different doctors. And no one could help me, Doc. You've made a believer out of me."

Like many of my patients, Helen came to see me for chronic back pain. A few weeks later, Helen's back pain was feeling much better, but it seemed she was not telling me the whole story. Helen, it turned out, could not taste or smell.

Two and a half years prior to her first visit, a virus had attacked her olfactory nerve leaving her without the ability to taste or smell. She visited many specialists about her condition, but none could help her. It had never dawned on Helen to disclose the loss of her senses because she thought chiropractic was only good for back pain.

It was through the faith of my other patients that Helen gained her faith. Over the course of a few weeks she had witnessed many incredible healings. A renewed hope began to stir inside of her. One day she finally revealed her secret to me. I examined her upper cervical spine and proceeded to deliver a series of specific chiropractic adjustments to that region.

Within two weeks, she had regained ability to taste and smell. Her faith in chiropractic is stronger than any patient I know.

Walter is the ultimate example of limitless healing possibility. Many years ago, Walter had open heart surgery. His life included routine visits to the cardiologist.

Six months prior to him becoming my patient, Walter experienced chest pains and was admitted to the hospital. During his hospital stay his condition worsened. He suffered a stroke and other complications. He received a complete and thorough examination by the head cardiologist at the best hospital in the state.

Walter was told the stroke had caused his heart to shut down. Everything was blocked. Nothing could be done. He was given a terminal prognosis and just weeks to live.

Being a man of hope, Walter sought second opinions from many doctors. All were coming to the same prognosis, until he met me.

When Walter first came to my office he did not tell me about his terminal prognosis. He was mainly concerned about the constant stabbing pain in the middle of his head, the visual blurriness and dizziness the stroke had caused. He was very concerned about not being able to walk without the use of a cane or do any gardening.

I immediately went to the top bone in his cervical spine and found it had severely shifted out of position. This was confirmed upon an upper cervical x-ray analysis.

I proceeded to give him a very specific adjustment to his atlas, the top bone to the cervical spine. What followed was truly a miracle in my opinion as his headache disappeared immediately. The following day Walter returned with no cane. He stated the blood flow had returned to his hands. He could actually feel his heart beating again.

It has been several months since Walter's first adjustment. I have met many of his family and friends who are now my patients. Walter's wife, Anne, whom his cardiologist told to plan for Walter's funeral, sees her husband still alive and healthier than ever. She believes Walter's recovery is nothing short of a miracle from God.

When I stepped forward in faith toward chiropractic I was able to see healings. And only when I was able to see healings did my belief in chiropractic grow. All we need is to begin opening the door to limitless healing possibilities with a little faith, even as small as a mustard seed.

"I assure you, if you had faith the size of a mustard seed, you would be able to say to this mountain, 'Move from here to there,' and it would move. Nothing would be impossible for you."
– Matt. 17:20 NAB

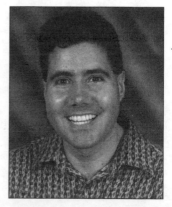

Gregory J. Sabatino, D.C.
Sabatino Family Chiropractic
Bridgeport, CT
203-333-4455
Dr. Sabatino specializes in family-based chiropractic.

CHAPTER TWO

COULD SUBLUXATION
BE HURTING YOU?

PART ONE

THE REAL TRUTH ABOUT HEALTH

By Dr. George A. Auger, D.C.

Our belief systems shape the way we perceive the world around us. We have political, economic, religious and health care belief systems. Our views and beliefs dictate how we act.

A belief is simply an interpretation we hold to be true.

At one point in our history, the world was thought to be flat. This was a predominant viewpoint among the wealthy, poor, noble and educated. Half a millennium ago, people also believed that the sun revolved around the earth. When Copernicus suggested our planet was not the center of the universe, people became very upset. Challenging prevailing beliefs inevitably generates resistance. However, new ideas introduced by courageous individuals eventually expand our awareness and bring us closer to the truth.

Eventually, we can accept new ideas and the world changes forever.

I believe we have an outdated "flat world" belief system when it comes to health care. A more accurate name for today's healthcare would be "sickness, symptom or disease care."

Why?

A number of people seek their doctors' advice only when they have a symptom or disease to be diagnosed and treated.

Many people believe health comes by treating disease and

pain. Most go through their lives carefree until their bodies break down, at which point they ask for help.

Treating your disease or pain is how you get healthy again, or is it? How did we ever adopt this interpretation of health care?

Television has been a powerful factor in shaping our belief systems over the past decades. Political, sociological, religious and health care belief systems have been formed based on what has been relayed to us through television.

How pure and accurate is the information coming into our households through this very potent and influential communication media?

Advertising sells. It is no different in health care. Pharmaceutical companies have promoted their health care belief systems since television became a household media. Could consumers be looking for options?

According to our current "flat world" mentality, people can take pills to rid symptoms and feel better. We are told this action can bring our body to a greater state of health. This has been aggressively sold to us over the years. However, is this true?

Health, by my definition, is not the absence of disease.

Does diagnosing and treating disease, really create *optimal* health and well-being? How about people who have lost their health? They have become sick or symptomatic. They are then successfully treated and returned to their pre-disease conditions. What if their pre-disease conditions are unhealthy?

These people would be no healthier now than prior to becoming ill.

People typically rest and eat better during an illness. This could raise their levels of health during their illnesses due to temporary healthy changes in lifestyle.

I believe the only way to reach optimal health is health enhancement including balanced nutrition, regular exercise, stress management, positive mental attitude, clean air, pure drinking water and good hygiene.

I feel a person is healthy when all the functions of the body are normally active. What part of your body is responsible for controlling and coordinating your functions? The answer is your brain.

The brain is encased in the skull and seemingly disconnected from the rest of the body. This is where the most intricate communication network known to mankind comes into play—the nerve system. The nerve system is responsible for carrying communication signals between the brain and the rest of the body. Unless your nerve system is able to carry these vital signals without interference, your optimal health and well-being could be compromised.

We are taught our level of health and wellness can be measured by how we *feel*. I feel this is one of the most dangerous misconceptions we have ever learned to accept.

Aches, pains and symptoms, in general, are not a definite indication of disease. Nor is the lack of symptoms an accurate indication of health. For example, suppose you stopped at a restaurant and ordered a hamburger. The sandwich happens to be spoiled. On the way home you begin to vomit and have diarrhea. You conclude that you are unhealthy and must somehow stop the vomiting and diarrhea.

In this situation are you actually unhealthy? No, your body is healthy as it begins to clear out (by vomiting and diarrhea) the poison (spoiled meat) from your system as quickly as possible. You would be unhealthy if you could not quickly clear the toxins from your body. The poison would then lock into organs and muscles creating the potential for dangerous health problems, possibly even death.

Smooth Path of Communication

Your brain communicates with your body via mental impulses sent over nervous system pathways within your spinal column. Communication interference can happen when a subluxation, or spinal bone misalignment, interferes with this pathway.

People with subluxations could be robbed of their vital abilities to optimally control and regulate their own bodies. This loss of optimal function could happen so slowly and subtly, people are unaware anything is wrong. In this all too common situation, the subluxation has existed, weakening and hindering the body's ability to properly function, for months or even years. At some point, long after the body has lost optimal functioning control, it will begin to give off symptoms or warning signs.

As an example, look at a person who has just been to the doctor's office for a routine checkup and was pronounced "healthy." On the way home he runs out of gas only a block away from the gas station. He pushes the car to the gas pump. While standing to catch his breath, he falls over with a heart attack. Just minutes earlier, he had no detectable symptoms and was pronounced healthy. In this example, he was unhealthy for a long time prior to his heart "giving out".

This scenario is not as rare as you may think. Many of us personally know of an individual who was seemingly "well" one day only to become "mysteriously sick."

Sickness, such as cancer, heart problems and internal organ problems, to name a few, do not happen overnight. However, sometimes it appears so because there are often no perceivable symptoms until the process has progressed to an advanced stage.

Symptoms, or a lack thereof, are an unreliable method of verifying your communication pathways are clear and your body is functioning optimally. This is why, I believe, a chiropractic checkup and correction of any spinal bones interfering with the nerve system are vital. Otherwise, you may not be functioning at your peak.

As we enter the new millennium, our ideas about the human body and its ability to heal itself are undergoing dramatic shifts. I see this opening possibilities for unprecedented health, vitality and longevity. I feel a move towards chiropractic care would revolutionize the American health care system. We would emphasize prevention rather than focusing on the treatment of illness, as is the current norm. As chiropractors, we are working together to increase chiropractic awareness to help people make informed, intelligent, responsible decisions concerning their own health and the health of their families.

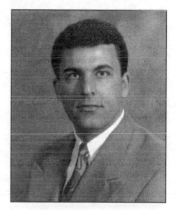

Dr. George A. Auger, D.C.
Auger Family Chiropractic
Greenville, SC
864-322-2828

PART TWO

The Body's Natural Medicine Cabinet

❦

By Dr. Ross D. Rutkowski, D.C.

If you woke up in a smoky room, would you pull the battery from the smoke detector to stop the noise and just go back to bed? Of course not.

In that same vein, why not develop new, more effective ways of dealing with health problems? Chiropractic care offers a powerful alternative that might enable patients to abandon medications in favor of healthier lifestyles.

How did our society become so dependent on medications? Perhaps we developed an inaccurate idea about wellness. Wellness does not have to mean dealing with a health crisis and surviving it. Rather, wellness could mean not having a crisis in the first place.

Many people believe health problems are caused by factors outside of their bodies, such as viruses and bacteria. As a result, they could also think cures come from outside, perhaps, in the form of medication. To me, this simply does not make sense.

Do you believe headaches are caused by lack of aspirin in the body? If not, then how can putting aspirin into the body be a solution?

I believe the body must be allowed to develop its own biochemical balance.

Consider the body's design. The body manufactures chemicals designed to meet our health and wellness needs. These include anti-inflammatories, pain-killers, anti-depressants and more. These chemicals help your body keep its balance, suppress pain, regulate your mood and live a healthy lifestyle.

But sometimes, your body's chemical makeup could get out of balance. Here are just a few examples that result in common health problems:

- Fatigue could cause extreme difficulties for patients, who may even find it difficult to get out of bed in the morning, much less live productive lives. Fatigue could be caused by slow metabolism occurring if the thyroid gland does not manufacture enough thyroxin. As a result, sufferers can grow overweight, regardless of their diet.

- Arthritis plagues men and women, young and old. This discomfort and joint pain could be caused by a chemical imbalance when the adrenal gland is not making enough cortisol. Taking powerful prescription drugs such as cortisone could cover the pain. However, one of the main effects of long-term use could be osteoporosis or thinning of the bones.

- Depression could be the result of hormonal irregularities and could include such depressive symptoms as problems sleeping and issues with appetite. Unlike once believed, depression is not simply an emotional problem. The limbic system is the area of the brain controlling activities such as emotions, physical and sexual drives and stress response. The activities of the limbic are so complex and important that disturbances could affect your mood and behavior.

To stop and reverse these imbalances, wouldn't it make sense to create conditions to allow the body to naturally correct its chemical balances?

The body's natural chemicals are manufactured by organs and glands. These organs and glands receive instructions from the brain. It orders your organs to make certain amounts of various chemicals and release them at particular times.

But sometimes, the instructions may not reach their destination. If the body's central nervous system is damaged or stressed, instructions from the brain could become garbled as they travel to the body.

To create a clear path of communication, any blockages of the nervous system known as vertebral subluxations, must be removed. This is where a chiropractor comes in. A chiropractor makes gentle adjustments to the spine. The goal of the adjustments is to align the spine back into its proper position. Once properly aligned, communication could flow clearer from the brain to the body again.

I believe the human body was designed to be healthy and well. It contains all the knowledge and wisdom necessary to heal.

Could we become victims of our fears when we lack faith, confidence and belief in our own innate intelligence? Could we fear something horrible could happen if we don't surrender and allow others to heal our bodies?

I believe this fear-based thought process could have us losing our objectivity and becoming slaves to fear instead of masters of health.

Chiropractic care could be a long-term solution to your health problems. Let's explore the reasons why choosing short-term, quick fixes might not be the best decision.

I believe some medications could interfere with the body's natural, effective defense mechanisms.

Vomiting provides a quick and efficient way for the body to expel harmful toxins. So why take medication to stop this process if you could be forcing the body to retain poisons?

Similarly, fever helps kill viruses and bacteria in the body. So why would you lower your body temperature, enabling those germs to thrive?

In my opinion pain medication does not take the pain out of the body, just the mind.

What's more, medications could actually cause dangerous and potentially fatal side-effects.

Adverse Drug Reactions, or ADR's, are a leading cause of death among Americans. In 1996, 108,000 Americans died from Adverse Drug Reactions to FDA-approved drugs properly administered by licensed medical professionals as reported by *The Journal of the American Medical Association.*

A CNN health report dated April 14, 1998 found serious Adverse Drug Reactions to FDA-approved drugs affected 6.7 percent of patients or 2.1 million people. In the study, serious Adverse Drug Reactions were defined as being hospitalized, having to extend a hospital stay or suffering permanent damage.

Even aspirin, which is taken by millions of Americans, could cause side effects. According to Rxlist.com, aspirin at doses of 1000 milligrams or higher per day could produce side effects including stomach pain, heartburn, nausea, vomiting, as well as, increased rates of gross gastrointestinal bleeding.

Instead of turning to drugs to change the chemical makeup of the body, why not take steps to allow the body to make these chemical alterations naturally?

Consider Amy who became my patient at age 8. When she first came into my office, Amy suffered from chronic and severe sinus infections and seizures. Because of her sinus infections, Amy had been taking antibiotics for approximately 10 days every month for the previous two years. Since the age of 14 months, she took high levels of Phenobarbital to control her seizures.

At her first visit, I adjusted Amy's spine. From that day forward, Amy never had another seizure. She has also never again taken antibiotics. That was eight years ago. Just recently she stopped taking phenobarbital.

By improving the health of Amy's nervous system, her body was able to better regulate its own chemistry. Therefore, she no longer needed outside medications to help her body achieve better health.

You could enjoy similar results. All it could take is a visit to your chiropractor to receive a specialized spinal check-up. Couple this with proper nutrition and you could be on your way to a medication-free life. You could no longer have to worry about the possible side-effects caused by pills. Plus, you could save significant money on medical costs.

Whole Food Eating

I recommend you choose a natural way of supplementation by eating whole foods. For example, if you are concerned about your calcium intake, eat broccoli. This vegetable could offer the perfect ratios of key vitamins to ensure good digestion and absorption.

The tomato is an amazing example of whole food nutrition. Considered to be one of the most perfect vegetables on earth, the tomato contains lycopene. One of lycopene's greatest qualities is its possession of extraordinary anti-carcinogenic and anti-tumor properties. Tomato anyone?

And don't think wellness means you will have perfect health. Even the healthiest person could occasionally develop a cold or suffer injury.

By visiting a chiropractor more often you could boost the immune system, which could promote a faster and more efficient recovery. Since my family started chiropractic care, we rarely experience sicknesses and have all been medication-free for 14 years.

The next time your doctor suggests medication, I recommend you take the following steps:

1) Ask the doctor why he or she believes you need the drug and how it will benefit you.

2) Ask him or her to detail the risks of taking this drug. Listen carefully whether he or she glosses over the risks or concerns you may have.
3) Ask if there are safer alternatives. Research alternative approaches and present them to your doctor.
4) Inform your doctor about any other medications you take, including over-the-counter drugs and herbal remedies. Ask about possible interactions.
5) Most of all, remember you are the boss. It's your body and ultimately your decision whether any possible benefits of the drug outweigh the possible associated risks.

As a reward for following these guidelines, you could have a lifetime of enjoying more energy, sleeping better and being sick less often.

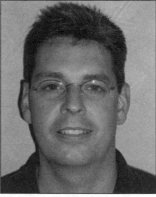

Dr. Ross D. Rutkowski, D.C.
Rutkowski Family Chiropractic Center
Somerset, MA
508-673-5400
Dr. Rutkowski specializes in
pediatric and family care.

PART THREE

SHIFTING THE PARADIGM OF HEALTHCARE

By Dr. Scott W. Poindexter, D.C.

Is subluxation of the spine being overlooked as a possible cause for sickness and disease? With a subluxated or misaligned spine, communication from the brain, through the spine, and out to the body's organs, muscles, and tissues could be greatly diminished.

Having completed my undergraduate degree in science, I already knew I wanted to be a doctor. I was just not sure what kind.

I was working as a recruiter for a major university when a student mentioned he was going to college to become a chiropractic doctor. At the time, I was under the care of a chiropractor. With my interest piqued, I conducted research and discovered chiropractic was a holistic healthcare profession which made perfect sense to me. Impressed with this non-invasive, whole-body healthcare approach, I knew my calling was to become a chiropractor.

My name is Dr. Scott Poindexter. I practice chiropractic healthcare in Lafayette, Colorado. My passion is changing the health paradigm in this country from medical "sick care" to chiropractic "wellness care."

Dangers of Drugs

Everywhere people look, magazines, newspapers, television and radio advertise the latest miracle drug. Could people be thinking optimal health and wellness could be found in a pill? As reported in the *Journal of the American Medical Association* on April 14, 1998, ADR's or Adverse Drug Reactions may be responsible for more than 100,000 deaths nationwide each year. In the December 16, 2002 issue of *AMNews*, the headline read, "Prescription drug abuse deadlier than use of illegal drugs." Did you know as reported by the Florida Medical Examiners Commission and the Florida Department of Law Enforcement, in Florida alone, prescription drug deaths exceed those from cocaine and heroin?

Why is That?

Parents are telling children to stay off drugs. Schools implement programs teaching children to "just say no." Yet, I believe our society, when it comes to children, promotes the use of medication for injuries, sicknesses and diseases.

In May 2001, the *New York Times* reported an 18.8 % increase for a total of $131.9 billion dollars being spent on prescription drugs in the United States. The World Health Organization ranks the United States at 37th on the world health index.

Is optimal health and wellness as simple as taking a pill?

I educate people that if the body is sustained with quality air, proper diet, right exercise *and* a healthy nervous system, the body could have amazing healing powers. I share with patients my belief that optimal healing comes from unobstructed communication from the brain, through the spine, and out to the body's organs, muscles and tissues.

Here is an example I use. Two people went to the same restaurant for dinner. Both indulged in the same high-sodium, high-fat meal. Only one person became sick with his or her body rejecting the food.

Which person is truly healthy? The healthy person, I believe, is the one who became ill. This individual's body is doing exactly what it was created to do, which is to rid the body of anything harmful.

Sadly, when people feel sick they may open the medicine cabinet and take something to stop the body's natural process of rejecting whatever is harming their systems. These people may have found temporary relief. They could have also suppressed the body's ability to remove toxins and decreased their levels of optimal health and wellness.

Consider for a moment a child running a temperature. Unless the temperature reaches a dangerous level, I believe the body should be monitored and allowed to heal naturally. Temperatures could be an important tool used by the body to fight germs, disease or illness. This could help strengthen the immune system.

When a child is given medication to reduce the body's temperature, is the opportunity to have a naturally strong immune system being compromised?

In this situation, I believe the chance for the child to experience optimal health and wellness throughout life could be lowered.

Medical care and surgery are invaluable for times of emergency crisis. I truly believe, however, if a person wants to live and maintain a life of optimal health and wellness that chiropractic must be the foundation. I think the paradigm needs to shift from medical "sick" or "crisis care" to chiropractic "optimal health and wellness care."

Wellness means experiencing physical, spiritual and emotional well-being, not just the absence of pain or disease. In my opinion, for optimal health and wellness to be achieved, the body's organs, muscles and tissues must function and regenerate 100% of the time!

Subluxation, or misalignments of the spine, could obstruct

communication required for the brain and nervous system to control the body's optimal function and regeneration. The health of the spine could degenerate if subluxations remain intact.

Physical, chemical and emotional traumas could cause subluxation and affect overall well being. These could start at birth and continue throughout life. Chiropractors work to correct subluxations, which could allow the body's "innate" healing process to reach optimal potential.

I believe innate intelligence is the internal force within the body which controls and regulates all functions through the brain and nervous system. When subluxations block innate intelligence, dysfunction could be created within the body.

In addition to educating my patients on attaining optimal health and wellness, I explain the important role that lifetime maintenance of the spine and nervous system play on living a quality life.

All too often, people take more pride in the care of their teeth, from getting braces to whitening them, than they do the very life force of the body, their nervous systems.

When the spine is adjusted and restored to proper alignment a patient may experience benefits such as increased energy, relief from allergies, enhanced sleep and improvement in overall health. My goal is to bring the body's physical, emotional and chemical aspects into balance each day and throughout life. I work with patients diligently encouraging them to keep their spines healthy and lead healthy lifestyles.

Subluxations cannot be felt. People without pain or symptoms of sickness or disease, and who look healthy, might believe their bodies to be at optimal levels of health and wellness. This may not necessarily be the case.

Consider a heart attack victim. Although he or she may have looked healthy and been symptom free, his or her heart could have been degenerating for years.

When a person has a subluxated spine, without correction,

he or she could be at risk. When the spine is subluxation free, the body's innate intelligence is allowed to function optimally without interference.

Health and healing come from within. The time has come for the healthcare paradigm to shift so people can experience true optimal health and wellness.

I believe the key to optimal health and wellness is simple. Get checked and adjusted for subluxations. This could aid your body's ability to replenish and regenerate. Work to keep your spine healthy throughout life with wellness chiropractic check-ups.

Optimal health and wellness is more than just living to an old age. It is living with a higher quality of life. Educating people is important. You can choose a personal health goal of having an optimal functioning spine and nervous system.

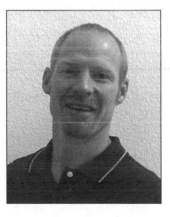

Dr. Scott W. Poindexter, D.C.
Indian Peaks Family Chiropractic
Lafayette, CO
303-664-0024

PART FOUR

WHY HAVEN'T I BEEN TOLD?

❧

By Dr. Francois Raymond, D.C.

What do you know about health care?

Can you imagine there is anything more? I invite you to sit down and be amazed by something right under your nose.

Often one of the biggest purchases we make, aside from real estate, is a new vehicle. When we purchase a vehicle we expect things to be in order and working at optimum level. After all, it's brand new with no structural damage, wear or tear.

We also expect complete and accurate instructions on its maintenance, in the form of an owner's manual and maintenance schedule from the manufacturer.

Those who have been careless in preventative maintenance, such as oil changes and tire rotations, know people only end up paying more in the long run. We can't possibly expect top performance when proper service has been neglected.

The same principles hold true for the human body. There is undoubtedly no more complex machinery than the body. It is a masterpiece.

The human body, with all of its wonderful structure and systems, is nothing short of a miracle. To imagine, in just nine months, it is possible for the body to grow from one single cell to a complex network of 100 trillion perfectly organized cells is mind boggling. All of this before you even enter this world!

This creative power is what I refer to as innate intelligence. It is the wisdom and ability of the body to grow and function in harmony with the environment.

The average heart beats 70 times a minute and over 100,000 times a day while pumping about 2,000 gallons of blood in a 24-hour period of time. In a 70-year lifetime, an average human heart beats more than 2.5 billion times.

Your spinal cord contains over 13 million cells transmitting electro-chemical signals. Your brain is made up of over 100 billion neuron cells that transmit signals to and from the brain at up to 200 miles per hour.

There are 206 different bones and over 650 muscles in your body. The body is miraculous in its ability to heal itself and regenerate cells. It is safe to say we are not the same person we were last year.

Just as a car needs regular tune-ups, the human body needs its systems checked and adjusted on a regular basis. Daily stress could cause optimal functions of the body to decrease if the body is not properly maintained.

Subluxations may cause a blockage in the spine reducing proper flow of nerve signals. You may not feel any pain or symptoms. Subluxations, left untreated, could cause the body to degenerate faster, further reducing the nervous system's ability to send uninterrupted signals throughout the body.

Care of the nervous system plays a monumental role in how our bodies regenerate. When there is interference on the nervous system, regeneration could slow down. When this happens, innate intelligence is not 100 percent and order becomes dis-order. Dis-order could lead to dis-ease.

As a doctor of chiropractic, I believe in a preventative approach to health through eliminating the nervous system interference by removing subluxations. Without interference, the body can do what it is naturally meant to do on its own. This is the chiropractic lifestyle and where chiropractic differs from mainstream medicine.

Why do some people have more confidence in a teaspoon of cough syrup or a pill than the life force that created them and the power regulating the universe?

When it comes to chiropractic care, some people may wait until crisis before taking action. This is unfortunate because subluxation could and often does occur without pain. It can take time for symptoms to appear.

What would happen if we cared for our cars in the same way? What would the outcome be of waiting until the tires were bald, the brake pads were completely worn or the oil ran out and all the signal lights were flashing before taking it into the shop?

Think about that! Now think of your body in the same way. Why wait for "check engine lights" or pain before having chiropractic maintenance?

Since the central nervous system is the governing system of the body, it has an impact on virtually everything. The nervous system is responsible for sending communications to the body's systems so they function orderly and properly.

When all is not well with the central nervous system, there could be communication breakdowns affecting the wellness of individual systems and the whole person. Subluxations could cause disorder and possibly allow dis-ease. Correcting subluxations could help prevent dis-ease and allow the process of wellness to begin.

By waiting for a signal of pain before seeing a chiropractor, a person could be neglecting what the nervous system is revealing. It is said only 10 percent of nerves register pain. The other 90 percent impact our lives by allowing our hearts to beat, lungs to breathe and organs to work properly keeping us alive. Your nervous system needs preventative care to avoid dis-order and dis-ease. By the time a pain signal occurs, the damage could be done. This is why I believe chiropractic check ups and adjustments, as part of your wellness routine, are so very important.

Regular adjustments could remove interference and allow properly functioning nerves to maintain optimal health. The body is a complete miracle! Let's count our blessings and do all we can to keep these amazing gifts functioning.

Remember the television program from the late 1970's "The Six Million Dollar Man?" If in the 1970's it cost $6 million dollars for two legs, arm and eye, what price would you put today on a whole body with all of its complex systems and miraculous capabilities?

Why haven't you been told this? Now that you know, tell the world! God bless you.

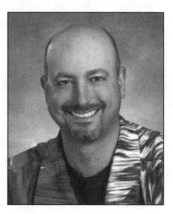

Dr. Francois Raymond, D.C.
Centre Chiropratique Raymond
Longueuil, Quebec, Canada
450-677-7411
chirosante@videotron.ca

PART FIVE

TOTAL LIFE CONDITIONING

~~~

By Dr. Joseph Denney, D.C.

Do you hit your alarm clock's snooze button three or four times?

Do you drag yourself out of bed with little passion for what life has to offer you?

Don't you want to wake up more excited with passion for life, rather than snooze through each day?

Prioritizing your health and wellness can be a good choice. Including chiropractic in your routine could help increase your health, wellness and total life conditioning.

Health is about choices! You make choices each day to move toward or away from health.

Once you commit to your health, a strategy can be created. You need to surround yourself with a team who has similar goals and the level of expertise to help you. Including a chiropractor on your team ensures someone is working for you to help unlock your potential for health.

The most important member of your team is you.

How do you 100% join your team? You make a commitment to have your spine checked and adjusted. Spinal adjustments remove nerve interference and open channels for your brain to communicate fully with all systems of your body.

Your brain could be one of your best coaches. Innately it

wants only the best for your body and desires for you to be healthy. It communicates this through your nerves. All winning teams need great communication. Would you say communication is a key to winning? Clear communication between your brain and your body is vital to health.

Olympic Health?

I spoke with an Olympic athlete who had his spine adjusted often by his chiropractor. In his quest for the gold medal, he had come to realize the necessity of training and performing at an optimal level.

This athlete's commitment to health was obvious, as was his desire to win a gold medal. He chose an approach that would help him achieve total body conditioning and go for a gold medal. He surrounded himself by a team with similar goals. His life actions and his choices were all geared toward reaching the gold.

Overcoming External Stress

In the real world, life can be challenging…to say the least. Have you read the paper or watched the news lately? Take some time off from the news. Start your day by reading what enriches your spirit. Follow these positive thoughts by awaking your body with light stretching and exercise.

Consider starting each day by *not* going back to sleep. Rather than reach for the snooze button, grab a book of positive quotes or spiritual literature. Make this a habit and start celebrating life with positive thoughts the minute you wake.

Living in Joy

You can make a commitment to live life with joy. I don't deny life can be challenging. Total life conditioning includes creating a strategy which nurtures and feeds the spirit every day. What feeds your spirit?

Could it be seeing as many sunrises and sunsets as possible?

How about being with family? Walking galleries or museums with great art and sculpture? Strolling a beautiful garden? Reading great poetry? Feeding your spirit can better equip you to overcome challenges with a positive, productive attitude.

Avoid starting and ending your day with violent TV or visual images that could negatively affect your spirit.

Part of my total life conditioning plan is to feed my spirit by traveling to Italy every year to visit my family. The food, the art, the clothes and the people are all amazing. Just walking around cities like Rome, Florence and Venice is enough inspiration to last a lifetime.

In the plan of life and health, passion needs to become apart of you. The Italians call it "La Dolce Vita," the good life.

Look at your life team. Have you surrounded yourself with others who share your values and your goals? Can you reach out to these people for help when needed? Can they reach out to you? Do you have a chiropractor on your team who helps you prioritize your health and make life conditioning possible?

It is my personal wish and my personal prayer for everyone to achieve optimal health including regular chiropractic care. By having a chiropractor on your team of life, you could increase the value of your health. Chiropractic adjustments, which remove vertebral subluxations, can help you to stay connected to your mind, body and spirit.

Like an Olympic athlete, train for your own Olympic event…Your life! Keep your gold medal health goal in sight. Recognize upfront you cannot do it alone. After all, Olympic athletes rely on a team and a strong support system from friends and family. Include yourself on your team. Honor your body and the gold medal of health can be yours.

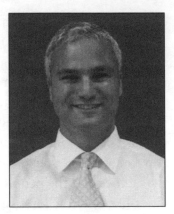

Dr. Joseph Denney, D.C.
Denney Chiropractic Center
Mount Laurel, NJ
856-439-9393
denneydc@aol.com

PART SIX

UNVEILING
THE TRUTH

❧

By Dr. Sima Goel, D.C.

Life is an expression of intelligence. How could we have a physical universe without some form of intelligence which created it? Similarly, how could the human body – which consists of trillions of cells, many organs and countless chemicals – function in harmony randomly?

Research shows the human body can eventually be reduced to dust and minerals. In this state, by my calculations, its elements are valued around $12. Yet, when we add water and intelligence, the body becomes priceless.

Consider the differences between a dead person and a live person. They share the same physical components: skin, bones, organs, blood, etc. The main difference is the live person has what chiropractors refer to as innate intelligence or energy flow. This innate intelligence or energy flow provides the properties of life: organization, respiration, reproduction, elimination and adaptation.

We cannot weigh or measure this energy flow with our five senses. But we can see the evidence of its power in every living human as people adapt to challenges. This energy flow transmits information through the body at amazing speeds via the spinal cord and nervous system.

Think about this. As you read this page, your eyes are transmitting images to your brain. Your brain is developing concepts. You might be listening to music. Your lungs are oxygenating red blood cells. Your stomach might be digesting food. All without any conscious effort. This illustrates just a few of the millions of functions your body performs each day, automatically and simultaneously.

If the body can organize its many functions so magnificently, shouldn't our focus be on optimizing this inner power?

If you wish to live life to the fullest, consider helping your energy to flow through your body properly.

When energy and information are transmitted properly from the brain through the spinal cord and nerves, the body is able to function optimally. The ability to self-heal could increase. When the spine is not cared for properly, the body could be more prone to injury.

Due to a lack of spinal hygiene and the stresses of life, the spinal vertebra could move out of their proper positions placing pressure on the nerves. As a result, people could be living with unnecessary physical limitations. Ignoring the damage could result in pain.

Your Internal Electrical System

For all the appliances in your home to function optimally, electricity must flow efficiently through the wiring. If a single circuit breaker in the fuse panel is tripped, and the circuit is broken, essential home appliances will not function.

It is the same with your nervous system. Doesn't it make sense that if the energy flow through the nervous system is blocked, the organ to which that nerve travels could suffer?

Even if you feel generally well, it does not always mean your body is functioning optimally. Some health problems could grow without your awareness.

In our society, when one of the thousands of potential diseases affecting the body arises, we are conditioned to seek the answer outside of our bodies. Should medication and surgery be our first options?

Some medications could block symptoms the body gives as warning signals when something could be wrong. Medication could numb symptoms forcing the body to scream louder and louder to alert us to problems. Certain medications could cause a host of negative side effects.

If the spine is not aligned properly, it could be difficult or even impossible for the body to solve its own problems. In looking for the root cause of health challenges, doesn't it make sense to start at the spinal column to be sure the nerves are bringing the proper energy to the organs?

As a chiropractor for 10 years, I believe there is a doctor within each of our bodies and our bodies' functions are guided by a healing intelligence bigger than any of us can imagine. I do not take any credit when my patients heal. The credit goes to the Creator of such magnificent, self-healing bodies.

Are You Healing?

Ask yourself questions that could guide your healing process. Do you want to fight symptoms of disease all your life, without addressing the underlying problem? Or do you want to heal the cause of your symptoms and optimize your health?

Just as some people turn to medication or surgery, others rely on lifestyle choices to maximize their health. Of course, eating properly and exercising are good for your body. But these behaviors alone could fall short of accomplishing your health goals if your nerve flow is compromised.

You might eat a healthy diet and exercise in an effort to lose weight. But, what if your stomach is not properly digesting food and preventing you from achieving a healthier weight?

I believe optimum spine and nervous system function equals optimum health. Visit a chiropractor for a check-up to determine whether there are problems with your nervous system. As my mother always said, "An ounce of prevention is worth a pound of cure."

If a subluxation is found, your chiropractor can help restore the flow of energy and healing within your body. Patients come into the office complaining of specific symptoms. Once the pressure creating the symptoms is relieved, I feel the body has a greater ability to heal.

As a mother, I encourage my children to follow healthy lifestyle habits such as eating properly, drinking lots of water and exercising. I help them understand how energy flows from their brains through their spinal cords to their nerves. I feel this helps my children understand their inner abilities to heal health challenges.

I write this chapter in loving memory of my father, who showed me throughout his life – even in his final moments – the greatest thought is the thought of joy, the greatest action is the action of love and the greatest word is the word of truth.

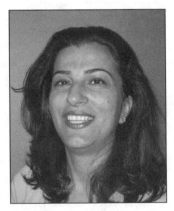

Dr. Sima Goel, D.C.
Decaria Square Family Chiropractic Clinic
Montreal, Quebec, Canada
514-344-6118
drsimagoel@bellnet.ca
Practice specializing in family and children

PART SEVEN

4+1 Essentials
of Life

By Dr. Martin LaPointe, D.C.

Life force flows through our nervous system distributing energy to cells and tissues in our bodies. In order to keep this force flowing and sustain life, we need food, water, oxygen and nerve impulse.

There is a fifth life essential we all need. That is love.

This fifth essential is most important for me. It is the glue holding everything together. I believe everything stems from love. After all, love brings life. Love makes life worth living.

Lack of self-love and love for others makes life unbearable. In fact, I firmly believe lack of love in one's life is the biggest cause of sickness and of death.

Health is a gift at birth. It should be maintained through our existence. Unfortunately, this can be a difficult task as few are given directions on exactly what we need for good health or how to maintain our bodies.

We are born with genetic health potential. I believe each generation could increase this potential provided people take care of themselves and lead healthy lives. This includes regular chiropractic care. My children have all been receiving regular chiropractic adjustments since birth. I began chiropractic care when I was 18 years old.

If people understood interferences to their health potential, they could avoid illness and keep health and wellness at the highest levels possible.

Like buying a car and servicing it regularly, we must service our bodies with regular chiropractic care. This helps alleviate negative interference which could damage our health and overall well-being.

People maintain their cars in accordance with manufacturers' recommendations. Doesn't it make sense people learn how to maintain their bodies using the recommendations of professionals including doctors of chiropractic?

Life Instructions

Food is the fuel needed for growth and reproduction of cells and tissues. Food, consisting of protein, fats and carbohydrates, is needed to survive. Without it, we will die. And, as the old saying goes, we are what we eat.

Poor nutrition leads to poor health. An imbalance could occur from consuming too much fat or too little essential fat. This could lower health potential.

Good nutrition means eating as many raw fruits and vegetables as possible. Eliminate processed foods. I recommend eating as many certified organic products as possible. This cuts down on the chemicals you may be unknowingly putting into your body.

Water is essential for good health. Did you know that your body is made up of 75% water? If you stop drinking water and eliminate other fluid intake, you will die in just a few days.

By drinking high-sugar or high-fat beverages, you could be jeopardizing your health potential. I strongly recommend drinking six to eight glasses of water every day. I advise my patients to drink fresh spring water instead of tap water, whenever possible. Again, this may help to cut down on chemicals you unknowingly place in your body.

Air, specifically oxygen, is another essential for life. Oxygen is used by every cell of our bodies. It is dispersed by the pulmonary (lungs) and the circulatory (blood) systems. Interference to these systems could impede oxygen travel, and significantly affect health.

To maintain these systems, and ensure your health, I recommend exercising aerobically for 30 minutes a day, at least four days each week. I also suggest regular weight training three times each week in addition to aerobic exercise.

This could mean setting the alarm early and getting up before the kids. It is a small sacrifice when you consider the increased health potential.

In addition, you are setting a good example for your children, who could increase the health potential of your family's next generation. This will hopefully continue for following generations.

Optimal nerve supply is the most commonly overlooked essential for achieving and maintaining good health. Electromechanical charges are transmitted by the brain through the spinal cord and nerves to the rest of the body. This is the life force keeping alive. All body functions are dependent on this charge.

Did you know every cell in your body has an electrical charge or potential?

Do you know what would happen if the nerves to your heart, lungs, stomach or bicep muscles were severed? The tissues and organs would cease to function.

Conversely, if you increased nerve transmission by decreasing interference, tissues and organs could be capable of optimal function.

The most common form of nerve interference is vertebral subluxation. This nerve interference can be very hard to detect without the help of a chiropractic doctor, because symptoms may not readily appear until 40 to 60 percent of nerve function is compromised. So subluxations could be present; and you may not be aware.

If your spine is subluxated, it is difficult to achieve your full health potential regardless of diet or exercise or even water and oxygen intake. I firmly believe nerve function is an essential for life and good health.

In my role as a chiropractor, I strive to remind my patients of these 4+1 essentials.

I stress eating well, drinking lots of water, exercising, breathing fresh air and aligning the spine to reduce or eliminate damaging nerve interference.

And, love every minute of life.

I tell my patients to love themselves, their bodies and those around them. Do this a little more every day. These are the 4+1 essentials my family and I live by. I encourage you and your loved ones to do the same.

Make sure to get regular spinal adjustments. This will remove nerve interference and allow the body to restore normal functions improving optimum health potential.

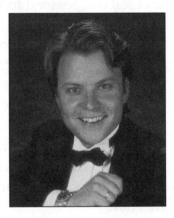

Dr. Martin Lapointe D.C.
Clinique Chiropratique St-Charles
Pierrefonds, Quebec, Canada
514-620-7229

PART EIGHT

FROM INJURY OR ILLNESS TO WELLNESS

❧

Dr. Perry Cammisa, D.C., BSc

During a visit to my home, a close friend who had suffered an injury told me he had turned to a chiropractor for help. My friend explained the adjustments used and how well they worked.

After his visit, which turned out to be life changing for me, I knew with 100% certainty that being a doctor of chiropractic was my calling. The following day, I changed my course of studies.

After graduating May, 1991 from Canadian Memorial Chiropractic College, I moved to the states and established my practice.

Medical doctors are referring a number of patients to chiropractors, as people seek options and alternatives from traditional care. I see patients from all lifestyles who have sustained injury through sports and various types of accidents. I also see people who have chronic headaches, back and neck pain.

In some cases, patients come to me as a last resort. Prior to becoming my patient, they might have been asked to undergo testing such as MRI's or CAT scans, therapies or medications without success.

Spinal Relationship

People think a headache is a headache and lower back pain is lower back pain. If there are problems with their organs, it is totally separate from everything else.

Educating people on the relationship between their spines and other parts of their bodies is a key element of chiropractic care. Working closely with patients to bring them from states of poor health, either from injury or illness, to optimal health or wellness is the goal of chiropractic care.

Although most people think the spine is straight, in reality, the spine has natural curvatures. When spinal curves are out of balance, the body could have difficulty functioning properly.

Think of the nervous system as a conduit for messages and information traveling from the brain to organs, muscles and other parts of the body. When the spine is under postural stress, messages and information can be interrupted or scrambled as they attempt to reach the intended target. This can be much like trying to communicate a message to someone over a cell phone with a bad connection.

In serving my patients, I focus on restoring motion to the spinal vertebrae allowing messages and information to flow properly. Chiropractic adjustments can facilitate the body healing itself with the goal of achieving optimal function.

Thinking of Health

It seems people have two thoughts on health. One is, "If it ain't broke, don't fix it". The other is, "If it is broke, fix it fast."

It is shocking to me. I believe many people take better care of their cars than they do their bodies. We could all be much healthier if we had easy-to-read, hard-to-ignore sensors like cars. Oil pressure low, oil light comes on. Temperature too high, temperature light comes on. Engine light on, stop the car!

The body has an amazing ability to adapt and accommodate for problems which have been going on for months or even years.

Humans have sensors. Many people ignore these internal sensors until their "engine light" comes on.

Internal sensors may be as simple as poor sleeping, digestive problems, muscle pain or headaches. Unfortunately, most people wait until problems disrupt their daily living before acting.

Some choose to mask these sensors with medication. Would you remove the battery from a smoke detector because the noise was irritating and ignore what caused the siren to go off? My observation is, in such a case of masking, the underlying issue could go unresolved.

Standing Healthy

Postural stress can be one of the sensors people ignore. How often do you think people experience postural stress?

Think about people working at computers five days a week. Can you imagine how much stress the spine endures?

Have you ever noticed when you get into your car to return home from work, you have to lower your car mirror and then the next morning you raise it again?

When leaving work, you may be slouching without realizing your condition. By the next morning, after your body has had time to rest, your posture may be a little better. Then, back to the office.

This cycle could repeat, sometimes for years, constantly subjecting your body to postural stress.

We live in a fast-paced society where people expect instant results. Sometimes I have to remind people they have been living with a specific problem for years. It might require time to resolve their problems with maintenance to keep them from returning.

Look at a person wearing braces. Did his or her teeth straighten over night? Is the spine any different?

Unfortunately many people think once pain is gone, they do not need to continue care. Yet, they continue subjecting their bodies to the same postural stress which caused the initial problems.

With consistent chiropractic care, people have the ability to maintain their body in a state of health. The nervous system has the opportunity to function optimally. This mindset is proactive, rather than reactive. It is preventative, rather than sick care.

Start Early

Although I help patients of all ages, my goal is be able to monitor patients' spinal health from youth. What is the reason? As patients grow, I believe chiropractic care can allow their bodies to maintain the highest level of health possible.

Do you know someone who has a "weather bone" from an old injury? When the weather turns or when the patient is stressed, the pain returns. The reason is the underlying problem was never fixed.

Many people can experience minor injuries and not even know it. Perhaps they have fallen off a bike or as children wrestled too rough with a sibling. Unless they have their bodies brought back into balance, they could experience aches and pains all their lives and not know why.

Do you remember the little red pills used in schools as an educational tool to show children areas missed while brushing their teeth? I feel as critical as the "red pill plaque check" is to dental care, so is a chiropractic subluxation check for correct posture.

Think of the body as a bucket which fills with water. The water increases as stress levels increase. Once at the top, the water begins to flow over. We can see the same in the body as stress levels increase producing more migraines, cold sores, acne, constipation, and so on.

Often, when patients come to my office, they are overflowing with problems. With each adjustment, I feel the water levels begin to recede. However, to keep the bucket from overflowing again, since we know stress is a large part of life, a wellness program needs to be implemented.

My goal is to improve quality of life with chiropractic care. Regardless of their ages, from babies to seniors, I want people to experience the remarkable difference chiropractic care can make in their lives.

Patients share this information with family and friends. By doing so, they could help more people find answers and alternatives to surgery or medication. Because of my work with patients and the incredible results I see, along with the love and support of my wife, I cannot imagine doing anything else more gratifying.

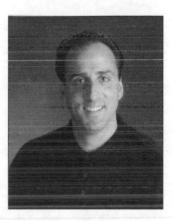

Dr. Perry Cammisa, D.C., BSc
Cammisa Chiropractic Health Center
Lisle, IL
630-778-9000

PART NINE

HEALTH TRUTHS AND MYTHS REVEALED

❦

Dr. Stuart Bernsen, D.C.

At age ten, my grandfather and I were sitting in the family station wagon waiting for my mother to return from running an errand. Although my grandfather was small in stature and a man of few words, he was big in wisdom and highly revered.

Unexpectedly, he turned to me and said, "Son, you should be a chiropractor."

With no explanation, my reaction was, "Okay, I will be a chiropractor".

Searching the library to find out what a chiropractor was, I found only two books on the subject. The first book was too technical. The second captured my attention as I read the first paragraph, "All living things, people, plants and animals have a force within that keeps it animated."

This was at the same time the movie *Star Wars* was as big as life. Although "the force" had nothing to do with *Star Wars*, after starting my practice, I realized the force relating to chiropractic care was far more powerful.

I ask my patients if given a choice, would they choose being healthy or sick. The answer is always healthy.

I ask, "What does health mean?"

The most common response I hear is "feeling good" or "not feeling any pain."

Health and wellness begin at conception. I believe within each fertilized egg lives all the wisdom needed for the body's creation. This wisdom, life force or innate intelligence is within every living human, animal, plant and organism. I view it as what created your body from a single cell to a multi-trillion cell organism in just nine months.

This wisdom or innate intelligence did not just randomly create your body. Would you agree it is possible that your body evolved in a specific order? Your brain, spinal cord and nervous system where among the first organs created.

As the body develops, the parts and systems form based on the body's priority. Since the lungs of a fetus are not required until after the baby leaves the womb, they are lower priority and therefore among the last vital organs to develop fully.

First Organs First

Your nerve system is your master system controlling and coordinating all of the other cells, tissues, organs and organ systems. No cell, tissue or organ in your body is separate from your nervous system. Rather, they are an extension of your nervous system.

To maintain optimal health and function, the brain must have an unobstructed path for sending messages down the spinal cord. A subluxation can place pressure on the spinal cord. When this happens, depending on the degree of subluxation, messages from your brain can become scrambled or blocked. The body can no longer fully communicate with itself.

Subluxations are silent, giving no indication of trouble. Unfortunately, most people believe they are healthy until they do not feel well.

Not until a lump or some other symptom arises do some people realize they could be dealing with disease. It is quite common for disease to progress over many years, without the person knowing.

Disease festers not with age, but with time. Let's use the example of twins who share the same genetic makeup with one subluxated at birth and the other not. When both twins reached age twenty, the one with subluxation could experience less health and vitality. This would be due to the amount of time the interference was in the body and not because of age.

Reaching Optimal Health

I believe people can reach optimal health with subluxations eliminated.

The role of the chiropractor is to remove subluxations. It is not to cure disease. Rather, we ignite the body's healing and communication abilities. With clear communication from the brain to the body, the healing process can occur. I believe as long as a person is healthy without subluxations, the body can take care of itself naturally.

There are many health myths. One is the role of genetics, which some people blame for their health conditions. Genetics may predispose us to experience certain traits and conditions. Genetics does not guarantee those traits and conditions will always be experienced.

How we live our lives could "turn on" or "turn off" expression of genes. For example, let us go back to the twins and assume they were predisposed to heart disease. What if one twin drank, smoked, did not exercise and had a poor diet while the other twin led a healthy lifestyle?

Which one of the twins is more likely to end up with heart disease?

The chiropractor's responsibility is to help people become aware of how to express their fullest potential, regardless of their genetic predispositions.

Is Subluxation Someone Else's Problem?

Subluxation can occur throughout life from stress, poor sleep, work habits, slips, falls, toxins and even the birthing process. Everybody can be susceptible to subluxation.

Subluxation is a natural part of life, and therefore not the problem. The real problem is the time during which subluxations remain in the body uncorrected. The longer subluxations remain in the nerve system, causing interference and decreased expression of life, the farther you could move from optimal health.

Subluxations controlled through regular chiropractic check-ups could result in less chance for damage.

Wellness is a proactive process, not a reactive event.

Chiropractors help the body optimize its natural healing abilities by removing subluxations. My purpose as a chiropractor is to help enable people to express 100% true health and wellness reaching their fullest life potential. This is my commitment to my patients and my family.

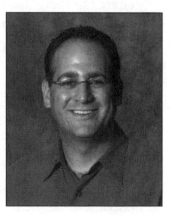

Dr. Stuart Bernsen, D.C.
Lifeline Wellness Center
Evanston, IL
847-475-4545
www.chirolifeline.com

PART TEN

EDUCATION IS KEY

∞

**By Dr. Cynthia Glendening, D.C. and
Dr. Andrew Gottlieb, D.C.**

Ours is a family practice based on education and the correction of subluxations. Our goal with our families is to have each member examined on a regular basis. Reducing and eliminating subluxations is critical to maintaining optimal health.

We believe that education with regards to reducing subluxations can optimize people's health and can improve their chances of living disease free lives. We define health as a state of optimal physical, mental and social well being, not merely the absence of disease. We believe some chronic conditions, like heart disease, diabetes and arthritis, begin to form in bodies long before presenting symptoms.

When optimally healthy you can fully express yourself through work, family hobbies, dreams and hopes. Chiropractic examinations, from birth on, could help you achieve this level of health.

We are all subject to daily stresses. We believe our abilities to feel good and overcome illness depends on unobstructed energy flow from the brain through the spinal cord and nerves out to the rest of the body. Subluxations, or misalignments of the spine, could reduce the vital flow of energy. Chiropractic adjustments may improve and restore the healthy flow of energy.

People tend to go to doctors only when they feel pain. What they don't realize is only a small percentage of the body's nerves send pain signals. The rest deal with body functions. As you are reading this book you are not thinking about your heart beating, your pancreas creating enzymes or your digestion. Your body is much more focused on overseeing those and many other functions than it is pain.

You could have subluxations and reduction of nerve flow long before you feel any pain or symptoms. Conversely, just because your pain or symptoms have disappeared doesn't mean the underlying subluxation is gone. You can't feel subluxations, only some of the effects.

A headache is a pain symptom, which could involve a subluxation. Usually, by taking an over-the-counter analgesic, the pain goes away. But have you ever wondered why they sell aspirin or pain relievers in bottles of 100 or more tablets? Could it be because the pills don't cure the cause of the headache? Can you see the importance of removing the cause?

Many people are under the impression it is bad to be sick. This is debatable. If your body reacts quickly and "flexes" its immune system, this is a positive response towards a diseased state.

Our children get sick as do other kids. The difference is when our children are sick, they get over it quickly. They are back to school the next day. The immune system depends on nerve flow. Doesn't it make sense to remove subluxations to increase nerve flow? This is the focus of chiropractic care.

We frequently demonstrate the need for chiropractic care with plastic demonstration spines located in various places throughout our office. You may be familiar with a demonstration spine from science class, health class or your chiropractor's office.

If someone comes in to our office with a sore shoulder, we'll ask how the injury happened. The patient may tell us of stopping suddenly on his or her bike and flipping over the handlebars. The patient may say he or she walked away without serious injury.

We'll grab one of the demo spines and use it to show the patient what happened when he or she hit the ground. We jiggle the demonstration spine to imitate the motion of peddling the bike. Then, flip the spine in the air simulating a body flying over handlebars. The demo spine crashes to the ground. This makes an excellent visual of how subluxations can actually occur. It's easy to see how twisting and falling can cause these misalignments.

Of course, that's an injury situation. Subluxation happens for all sorts of reasons. Poor posture, lifting injuries, weekend warrior activities and sitting in front of computers are all activities which could cause subluxation. Our bodies tighten up under stress, which could cause subluxation. It's amazing how much a chiropractic adjustment can improve mood as well as physical well-being.

There are lots of children who are patients in our practice. We have two youngsters of our own, ages five and eight. It often seems kids 'get' the idea behind the need for chiropractic care quicker than their parents. Could it be because they haven't been exposed to as many years of media or advertisements as their parents?

Our children have been known to tell their playmates with colds that the playmates need adjustments. We've explained to our children blocked nerve flow compromises the body and the immune system. They understand this problem and a chiropractic adjustment is often a resolution.

Chiropractic focuses on a very basic principle of allowing the body to heal from above-down and inside-out.

Ideally, we like to start check-ups as soon after birth as possible. When you consider the pressure placed on a child's head and neck area during birth, it's not surprising subluxations could occur. The newborn body does not have the musculature to combat the force applied during the birthing process, thus the body could react by creating subluxations.

Our own children have received chiropractic care and adjustments since the day they were born. It's no coincidence they have not taken any antibiotics or drugs for colds, earaches or the many other typical childhood illnesses.

We have established a network of allopathic doctors and other medical professionals. If one of our patients needs blood work, an MRI or to have a broken bone set, we refer him or her to the appropriate professional for specific tests or treatment. We support the medical treatment with chiropractic care.

In return, other doctors and medical professionals refer for correction of subluxations in their patients who have not responded to drug therapy or surgery.

We take pride in the quality of our practice and our patients. Our patients are people who truly want to be helped and are willing to work with us to improve their health. We want people to join our practice because maintaining optimal health is a top priority.

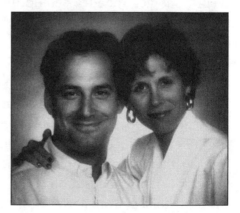

Dr. Andrew Gottlieb, D.C.
Dr. Cynthia Glendening, D.C.
Eagle Chiropractic, P.C.
Uwchalnd, PA
610-458-7777

CHAPTER THREE

CAN CHILDREN HAVE SUBLUXATION?

PART ONE

A SECOND CHANCE AT LIFE

~~~

By Dr. Richard Statler, D.C., D.I.C.C.P., C.C.S.P.

The numbers are alarming. An article released by the California Department of Developmental Service revealed the number of children with autism increased by 273 percent between 1987 and 1998. In 2001, an all-time, one-year record number of cases were diagnosed in California. Today, in some parts of the United States, 1 out of every 400 children is autistic.

According to research published in the book *Vaccines: Are They Really Safe and Effective?* by Neil Z. Miller, "In 1943, the well known child psychiatrist, Leo Kanner, announced his discovery of eleven cases of a new mental disorder. This condition soon became known as autism. These first cases of autism in the United States occurred at a time with the pertussis vaccine was becoming increasingly available. By the 1950's and 1960's, parents from all over the country were seeking help for their autistic children. The growing numbers of children suffering from this new illness directly coincided with the growing popularity of the mandated vaccination programs during these same years."

Miller continues, "When the United States ended the war and occupied Japan, a mandatory vaccination program was established. The first autistic Japanese child was born in 1945. Europe received the pertussis vaccine in the 1950's; the first cases of autism began to appear there in the same decade. In England the pertussis vaccine wasn't promoted on a large scale until the late 1950's. Shortly thereafter, in 1962, the National Society for Autistic Children in Britain was established."

What can be more devastating for parents than to learn that their child is autistic? The severely debilitating neurological disorder, which affects social and language development, can be extremely difficult to treat. Often, a meaningful conversation or even eye contact is impossible.

In the more profound cases, children can spend their entire lives in isolation, with no response to words, actions or activities of people around them. As a result, parents are often advised to put their autistic children in institutions and get on with their own lives.

A press release from www.vaccineinfo.net, which can be viewed at the time of writing at http://vaccineinfo.net/issues/mercury/autismHg.shtml, announced the law firm of Waters & Kraus was the first to file a lawsuit alleging a mercury preservative, thimerosal, in children's vaccines caused neurological damage to an infant who was eventually diagnosed with autism. They have been joined by several other firms and their clients.

Lead attorney in the case, Andy Waters, announced his firm had possession of a previously unreleased confidential report authored by the Center for Disease Control scientists that studied autism as a potential neurological injury caused by mercury in children's vaccines.

According to Waters, the confidential version of the study states an exposure to more than 62.5 micrograms of mercury within the first three months of life significantly increased a child's risk of developing autism. The currently recommended course of vaccines could expose an infant to 75 micrograms of mercury in the first three months of life. The study reported a 2.48 times increased risk of autism, meaning exposed children were more than twice as likely to develop autism as children not exposed.

According to the release from Vaccineinfo.net, the United States courts have generally upheld that a relative increased risk of 2.0 or higher is sufficient to substantiate that a given exposure caused disease. In the case of Cook v. United States, 545 F. Supp. 306, at 308 (Northern District California, 1982) the Court stated, "In a vaccine case, a relative risk greater than 2.0 establishes that there is a greater than 50% chance that the injury was caused by the vaccine."

According to *The Vaccine Guide* by Randall Neustaedter, OMD (North Atlantic Books) chemicals used in the preparation and preservation of vaccines could include mercury, formaldehyde and aluminum.

Neustaedter goes on to report "a 1994 survey of 159 doctors' offices by the National Vaccine Information Center revealed that only 18 percent of doctors said they make a report to the government when a child suffers a serious health problem following vaccination."

Former director of the FDA, Dr. David Kessler, is quoted as to saying, "Only about one percent of serious events (adverse drug reactions) are reported."

According to Neil Miller, "In the last few years, more than $1 billion had already been granted for thousands of injuries and deaths caused by mandated vaccines. Numerous cases are still pending. Awards were issued for permanent injuries that included learning disabilities, seizure disorders, mental retardation, paralysis and numerous deaths, including many that were initially misclassified as sudden infant death syndrome (SIDS)."

I highly recommend reading both *The Vaccine Guide* and *Vaccines: Are They Really Safe and Effective?*

I cannot foresee how the Vaccine Compensation System for vaccine-injured children can support the families of these children whose costs could be millions or billions of dollars in ongoing lifetime medical care. In my opinion, the system is so difficult to qualify for and navigate through that many people may not be compensated for damage to their children.

While the battle against the harmful effects of vaccinations continues, the question remains: How can we best help the children who might have been damaged already?

Historically, autism has had a bleak prognosis. Fortunately, chiropractic could present a hopeful perspective.

The focus of chiropractic for children with disabilities, regardless of the symptoms, is to correct and manage the subluxations that block proper nerve flow. When the nerve interference is removed, miracles could become possible. Early diagnosis and intervention is critical and may help maximize children's potentials. The following real-life stories demonstrate how chiropractic can offer autistic children a second chance at life.

When seven-year old Gavi was first carried into our office, he seemed unreachable. He could not speak, focus, walk or even stand on his own. His parents were advised to put him in an institution because "the child would never be able to have any meaningful communication with anyone." After two years of regular adjustments, Gavi has changed the predetermined course of his life. While boys with his genetic condition typically get worse with time by becoming aggressive and losing all communication skills, Gavi is making amazing progress. He talks, walks, runs and plays. He is the most loving person you can imagine!

Like many other autistic children, David was constantly screaming and making flailing motions with his body. He had no sense of other people's personal space, which made it very difficult for his parents to take him out in public. After only two months of adjustments, he is a completely changed child. David can now sit and wait his turn when he comes into the office, maintain eye focus, vocalize his needs and interact with others. His parents are overjoyed with this transformation.

Another challenged child, Tommy, used to constantly bury his entire index finger up into his nose. Although this was diagnosed as a behavioral problem, it appeared that the bones in his skull were jammed and he was trying to relieve the pressure. As I worked with the cranial bones around his eyes, forehead and the bridge of his nose, Tommy's problem went away because we found and corrected the cause.

Courtney had Pervasive Developmental Delays (PDD). She was still in kindergarten when the doctors began preparing her parents for the worse. It was possible that by fifth grade, Courtney would need spinal surgery because her severe scoliosis was rapidly growing worse.

Courtney was already at nineteen degrees when she started chiropractic care. If we could have just stopped her scoliosis from progressing, that alone would have been a huge win! In the first six months of regular adjustments, her scoliosis reduced by five degrees. Then, it improved by five more degrees within the next six months.

The doctors were very impressed and told Courtney's parents to "continue using the brace." The irony was the child was so uncomfortable in the brace they never used it!

Courtney has experienced some profoundly positive changes in her life since she began her care with us three years ago. Today, she is a much happier and higher functioning child.

Angelo walked into my office with his mother, a registered nurse, on a particularly busy morning. He was constantly making loud noises. Seeing his mother's obvious distress, I started the consultation right away, before looking at the chart. It appeared that Angelo was the ideal candidate for chiropractic adjustment.

I introduced Angelo's mother to another patient, about the same age as Angelo and with a similar autistic condition. The little boy was sitting on his mother's lap, humming softly and showing remarkable signs of love and affection. Seeing this beautiful bonding moment gave Angelo's mother a sense of hope.

While the mothers had a chance to get acquainted, I started

working on Angelo's skull and after a few minutes he obviously felt better and stopped screaming.

After Angelo and his mother left the office, I learned that the appointment was originally scheduled for the mother, not the child. When I called to apologize about the misunderstanding, Angelo's mother, who is a registered nurse, could not have been happier and was looking forward to her son's next adjustments with us.

As a second-generation chiropractor, I am dedicated to the nerve system health of children with disabilities. My mission is to educate and adjust as many families as possible toward optimal health through a very specific, natural corrective chiropractic approach. Education is as important as the care itself because to understand autism and overcome their fears, parents need both information and hope. By talking with other people who have similar experiences, families dealing with autism learn they are not alone.

Medical and other doctors visiting my office often ask for a precise list of disabilities of the patient. More often than not, I have to check my files to provide them with this information. Instead of concentrating on a specific disorder, I am checking and adjusting my patients for subluxations.

When I look into the eyes and soul of my patient, I see a perfect little being trapped in an imperfect body. By removing nerve interference caused by subluxations, chiropractic adjustments help restore the life force in this body. This helps the body begin to restore itself to better health and wellness. Chiropractic offers autistic children a chance to realize their true potential, and helps close the gap between their world and ours.

Recommended reading and websites for parents and those concerned about vaccinations:

- *Mothering* Magazine November/December 2002 issue www.mothering.com
- *Vaccines: Are They Really Safe and Effective?* Neil Z. Miller

with forewords by Dr. George Schwartz, MD, and Dr. Harold Buttram, MD

- *The Vaccine Guide: Risks and Benefits for Children and Adults* Randall Neustaedter, OMD
- *Vaccines, Autism and Childhood Disorders: Crucial Data That Could Save Your Child's Life* by Neil Z. Miller
- www.909shot.com which is the website for the National Vaccine Information Center, a parent-sponsored group which lobbies for safer vaccines and freedom of choice legislation.
- www.thinktwice.com which is a site containing articles about vaccines and a list of worldwide vaccination support groups.
- www.vaccineinfo.net which has updates on legal issues and media coverage pertaining to vaccines. This site is operated by a Texas-based consumer group called Parents Requesting Open Vaccine Education (PROVE).

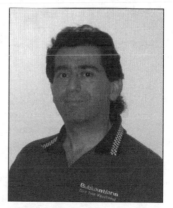

Dr. Richard Statler, D.C., D.I.C.C.P., C.C.S.P.
Statler Chiropractic
Huntington, NY
631-424-BACK (2225)
www.statlerchiropractic.net

Dr. Statler specializes in family, pediatric, sports and special needs care.

"Tis curious that we live only as deeply as we believe."
– Thoreau

PART TWO

WHAT IS HEALTH?
YOUR HEALTH PATH

❧

By Dr. Robert Martines, D.C.

Health is more than the absence of disease. It is the presence of abundant physical, mental, emotional and spiritual well-being.

Health is not a destination, rather a life-long, glorious journey. True health is sustained by consistently making wise choices that keep us on a path of wellness.

In Robert Frost's poem *The Road Not Taken,* he wrote eloquently about choosing a life path "two roads diverged in a wood, and I — I took the one less traveled by, and that has made all the difference."

Americans may be currently on a path of poor health, a path they didn't choose. Do you wait until your body gets very sick before you seek attention from a health care provider?

Is the current prevailing health care system, in reality, a sick care system?

Source of Sickness

Sickness is usually blamed on a "bug." These "bugs" could actually be bacteria or viruses and are generally treated with antibiotics until we feel better. Once we feel fine, we are pronounced well or healthy.

Can you expect a bountiful harvest from a garden by only

exterminating the bugs with insecticides when bugs appear? Probably not; clearly, much more would need to be done. Things like enriching the soil, consistent watering, pruning and so forth. In short, a vigilant tending of a garden is required to reap a bountiful harvest.

Abundant physical, mental, emotional and spiritual well-being requires vigilant tending. Most importantly, well-being requires first you choose a path of wellness rather than be passively blown like a tumbleweed down the path of illness.

If you fail to make this choice, you could end up like so many in our retired population, physically decrepit, overweight, lethargic, overmedicated and hopelessly depressed.

Don't you and your family deserve better?

You possess more intelligence, more will and more choices than a tumbleweed; so choose the path less traveled. Choose the path to better health.

What Can You Expect?

How does someone get on the well-being path and stay there?

It all starts by developing a powerful vision of what true health is for you. See yourself as vibrant, strong, compassionate, cheerful, loving and relaxed. Next, visualize what it takes to make health and well-being a part of your every day life.

For me, these are the first steps in determining a path that could bring physical, mental, emotional and spiritual health in abundance.

This visualization process is much like the one used by famous artist Michelangelo who, I am told, did not see the massive crude marble when creating his celebrated sculptures. Instead, he saw the beautiful sculpture inside and chipped away at the marble to reveal his vision.

This can be easily related to health. Visualize your ideal health and healthy habits. Then chip away at everything not a part of the picture.

As you journey this path to health and well-being, you will make choices necessary to ensure good health. These choices may include reducing unnecessary stress, getting enough rest, exercising regularly and eating balanced, nutritious meals and snacks.

The next critical step is to understand health is an inside job. It is important to understand our physical, emotional, mental and spiritual well-being depends on optimal nerve system function.

Our brain and the energy flow from it to every organ are paramount. I have been told a person could live perhaps 40 days without food, four days without water and four minutes without air.

However, a body can not live many seconds without nerve flow.

Take a minute to consider this: Today, your heart will beat more than 100,000 times pumping into blood vessels, which could wrap twice around the Earth. You don't have enough blood to cover this job all at once. Your nervous system must constantly move blood from one area to the next.

If we tried to duplicate what your brain does to run your body, I believe it would require a computer the size of Texas and as high as the Empire State Building being continuously cooled by the entire Hudson River.

Your brain and spinal cord (your super computer) is constantly "on" to sustain life, 8,760 hours a year. To put this runtime into perspective, consider a car driven 8,760 hours at 65 MPH would travel 569,400 miles in a single year!

Do you feel like your body has driven that many miles in the last year? It might if you haven't chosen and stayed on the path of health.

It's More Than Eating Right and Exercising

Many people still feel stressed, fatigued and disconnected despite proper exercise and diet. While diet and exercise certainly contribute to good health, optimal health cannot be obtained until interferences to our nerve flow have been removed.

These interferences are referred to as spinal misalignments or subluxations. By detecting and correcting these subluxations, the nerve flow from the brain to the body and from the body back to the brain can be restored.

Spinal alignment allows you to reconnect more completely to your internal power source — your nerve system. When your spine is aligned and your central nerve system is functioning without interference your body could function at its optimal level. Healing, on many levels, could occur in this way.

Nervous system interference could be devastating to one's health. Correcting interferences can be powerful. I believe the clearest example of this principle comes from an infant I adjusted several years ago.

Wellness Starts at Birth

Three-day-old Kelly Anne had been crying non-stop since her birth. A battery of tests at the hospital could not find the culprit for her endless crying. Yet, the newborn refused to breastfeed, drink from a bottle or even sleep.

At the time, I specialized in musculoskeletal /sports injuries, and was not sure if, or how, I could help this troubled newborn.

The parents persisted. I reluctantly agreed to see Kelly Anne. When she arrived at my office, I was shocked to see the parents carrying a small, beet-red body rigid with flexed arms and hands. The newborn baby's cry was ear piercing. I will never forget the sight or the sound of young Kelly Anne in obvious terrible discomfort. I knew immediately something was very, very wrong.

Upon examination, I found the top bone (the atlas bone) subluxated putting pressure on the nerve supply in her spinal cord. I explained this to her parents. I delivered an adjustment with faith and pure intent.

Kelly Anne's color went from red to pink. Her painful cry

settled into a baby's soft whimper. Her rigid body finally relaxed.

As her parents took her out to the car, our office staff and patients, who had witnessed Kelly Anne in such pain when she entered earlier, wanted to know what had happened.

Before I could explain, Kelly Anne's parents came back into the office with joyful smiles and whispered, "She's asleep."

From that day forward, I never questioned the power of an adjustment.

I believe adjustments are needed for total health, and absolutely essential for optimal nerve system function. This is why people like Tiger Woods, Lance Armstrong, Mel Gibson, country music legend Lee Greenwood (*God Bless the USA*), baseball's great and Hall of Famer Joe Morgan, sports stars, and Olympic champions receive chiropractic care. They realize the importance of 100% nerve flow. In my opinion, these people have chosen the path to health. They understand chiropractic care is an integral part of the health path.

Recently, the World Health Organization (WHO) rated the United States of America 37th in overall health immediately behind Costa Rica (36th) and just ahead of Slovenia (38th) and Cuba (39th).

It is hard to believe a country as advanced as the United States is, in my opinion, lagging so far behind when it comes to the health of its citizens.

As individuals, we could make the decision to change this and start on the path to good health joining 25 million chiropractic patients.

If you are not on a path to better health, make the commitment to change today. If you are already on this path, make a commitment to take your health to the next level and include regular chiropractic care.

Reward yourself and others for choosing the path less traveled, it will make all the difference. Remember, your life is a gift from God. What you do with your life is your gift back to God.

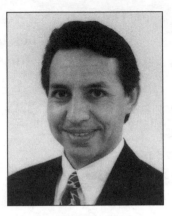

Dr. Robert Martines, D.C.
Chiropractic Health Center
Campbell, CA
408-378-1881
www.drrobertm.com

PART THREE

WHAT ARE YOU CHOOSING FOR YOUR CHILD?

❧

By Dr. Robert Stephen Watson, D.C.

He can't sit still. He can't focus on the task at hand. He is impulsive, hyper and hard to control.

Sound familiar? These are symptoms of Attention Deficit Disorder (ADD) and Attention Deficit Hyperactivity Disorder (ADHD), which have become increasingly common diagnoses for children in today's society.

Children with ADD display a specific set of characteristics. These include being easily distracted, failing to pay attention to detail, making careless mistakes, losing and forgetting things along with difficulty focusing attention on learning something new.

Children with ADHD seem to be always in motion. Sitting still may be a difficult task. They may fidget, squirm in their seats, be unable to wait their turns, talk excessively and feel restless.

Not every child who displays symptoms of ADD or ADHD is living with the disorders. Gifted children can display these behaviors and could be misdiagnosed.

The main medications being used to treat ADD and ADHD are methylphenidate and amphetamine. According to the United States Drug Enforcement Agency (DEA) at www.deadiversion.usdoj.gov/schedules/schedules.htm it reports that other names for methylphenidate and amphetamine are

Ritalin®, Adderall®, and Dexedrine®. The United States DEA has determined these drugs to be Schedule II controlled substances. What does a Schedule II controlled substance mean?

According to the United States Drug Enforcement Administration's web site at http://www.usdoj.gov/dea/agency/csa.htm, "The Controlled Substances Act places all substances that are regulated under existing federal law into one of five schedules. This placement is based upon the substance's medicinal value, harmfulness, and potential for abuse or addiction. Schedule I is reserved for the most dangerous drugs that have no recognized medical use, while Schedule V is the classification used for the least dangerous drugs."

Could this mean the Schedule II drugs being giving children are medications with the highest degree of harmfulness and potential for abuse or addiction?

Drug Enforcement Agency data also states methylphenidate "is an amphetamine-like central nervous system stimulant with properties that are similar to cocaine."

In addition, a wide range of side effects have been reported from these ADD and ADHD prescriptions such as headaches, mood swings, loss of appetite, irritability and sleeplessness.

According to the National Institute on Drug Abuse, adverse effects of methylphenidate could include high body temperature, irregular heart rate, cardiovascular system failure, fatal seizures, hostility or feelings of paranoia.

Do these drugs really address the root cause of the problem? Are children being taught to deal with their problems through drugs or medication, rather than seek out other solutions?

Plus, by taking these medications, are children made to deal with possible side effects or addictions?

Some of my patients have chosen a more natural solution to treat the root causes of their children's attention disorders. Through chiropractic care, these children have seen dramatic improvements in their behaviors, as well as their outlooks on life.

Seven-year-old Brenan was one such child. After an auto accident, his family took him to see the pediatrician. This doctor performed a two-minute examination. She asked Brenan to touch his toes and do jumping-jacks. When the boy accomplished these simple tasks, he was pronounced uninjured by the pediatrician.

At a prior appointment, Brenan's parents had asked the doctor about his problems with inattention and hyperactivity. The pediatrician recommended prescription drugs to address these behavioral issues.

Unhappy with the idea of giving their child such powerful psychoactive medications, and uncomfortable with the quick pronouncement he had not suffered damage in the car accident, Brenan's parents brought him to my office for a spinal health checkup.

During the examination, Brenan was almost unable to sit still long enough for a scan. He instead followed his impulses to move about the examination room, jumping, hopping and loudly seeking attention from his parents.

The evaluation revealed several severe subluxations, so we embarked upon a regimen of chiropractic care. After just one adjustment, his parents were thrilled to see Brenan calming down. He experienced improved sleep, as well as better digestion.

When people hear this story, they often express disbelief. Our society preaches that ADD and ADHD result from a chemical imbalance, so how could adjustments to the spine improve children's behavior?

The answer is simple. Irritations to the nervous system could directly cause behavior problems. When children suffer from subluxations, or misalignments in the spine, it could block mental impulses that travel to their vital muscles and organs. These blockages may prevent them from adapting to change effectively.

In essence, chiropractors seek to enhance each patient's neurological function by maximizing communication of the central nervous system. Neurological dysfunctions may be reflected in behavior.

For instance, suppose a child eats a candy bar or drinks a soda. The body needs to adapt to those changes. But what if there is a block in the spinal column which hinders communication between the brain and the stomach? The result could be an imbalance in biochemistry, which may be caused chiefly by misalignments in the spine. So this child might experience bad digestion, as well as extremely hyperactive behavior.

Subluxations: A Wide Range of Causes

The first subluxations can result from the birth process. As the child learns to crawl, walk, run and ride a bike, he or she will invariably suffer falls and minor injuries. Each of these incidents could result in a subluxation.

To improve children's spinal health, parents could choose to take their children to chiropractors for thorough spinal evaluations. If subluxations are detected, a course of gentle adjustments will be recommended until correction is achieved. At that time, wellness care will help maintain the correction.

Beyond adjusting these subluxations in the spine, parents can take other steps to help children with ADD and ADHD.

The first step is proper nutrition. Just as drugs have a powerful effect on the body's systems, so does food. If your child displays symptoms of ADD or ADHD, try removing the following foods from his or her diet: chocolate, flour, wheat, milk, eggs, food coloring, additives and flavors, along with corn, sugar and other forms of sweetener.

I recommend my patients to stay away from dairy products, which could be rife with additives, hormones and steroids. Consider using rice milk as an alternative to cow's milk.

Next, take steps to remove emotional stressors from your children's lives. While some stress is unavoidable, children can deal with situations better if given greater access to their parents. I frequently advise my patients' parents to spend as much quality time as possible with their kids. I believe this contact can greatly reduce the symptoms of ADD and ADHD.

Finally, make sure your children get enough exercise. This creates several benefits. First, children prone to hyperactivity need positive ways to burn off their excess energy. Sports and exercise programs can give them a great outlet to expend extra energy while building self-esteem.

Exercise also creates physical benefits. One specific exercise, called the cross-crawl pattern, is particularly useful for children with ADD or ADHD. For more information on the effectiveness of crawling to help with ADD/ADHD, I suggest a book entitled *Stopping Hyperactivity: A New Solution* written by Nancy O'Dell, Ph.D., and Patricia Cook, Ph.D., (1997, Avery Publishing Group).

With a program of proper nutrition and exercise, plus good spinal health, ADD and ADHD patients could experience great improvement. Once we remove the irritation to their nervous systems, this holistic approach could help children become more efficient users of their energy. Their organs are able to work in unison, putting their bodies and muscles back into balance. Plus, by smoothing the way for nerve transmissions, children's bodies can work at higher levels – both mentally and physically.

Children are our most precious resource. Let's all commit to healing their entire bodies, not just removing symptoms. Let us create a state of wellness that could last well into adulthood. As parents, our choices for our children can last their lifetime. Remember, as the twig is bent, so grows the tree.

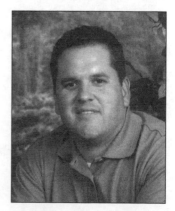

Dr. Robert Stephen Watson, D.C.
Mountain View Family Chiropractic, LLC
Oro Valley, AZ
520-818-7788
rswatson@yahoo.com

PART FOUR

Silent Subluxations

❦

By Dr. Craig T. French, D.C.

Blurry-eyed and fumbling, you're awakened from sound sleep by the horrific cries of your two-year-old child. You stumble into his room, feeling helpless as you lift your tear-soaked son out of his crib. He is feverish, pulling on his ears screaming, "Hurt, Mommy, hurt!"

You bundle him up and rush him to the hospital emergency room, which is the only place he can receive medical care at that late hour. Once there, you are directed to a hard plastic chair. You rock your feverish, miserable child as you wait for hours to see a doctor. You try in vain to calm him amid the chaos of the waiting room, where adults and children sit bleeding, coughing and crying.

Too many parents face this grim scene, as their youngsters endure a painful string of ear infections throughout childhood. Whether you rush to the emergency room in the middle of the night or wait for hours to be "squeezed in" at the pediatrician's office, the results are often the same: a prescription for antibiotics. This in turn may create unpleasant side effects and lead to drug-resistant bacteria, which could cause more serious diseases.

As parents, we would do anything to provide comfort and peace for our children. What too many parents do not know, however, is a dose of prevention might prove far more valuable to their children's health than all of the antibiotics in the world. Instead of relying on drugs to treat our already-ill children, wouldn't it make sense to take steps and stop them from becoming sick in the first place?

To have a healthy body, your central nervous system – which is made up of the brain, spinal cord and nerves – must be working well. Sometimes a misalignment of the spine, also known as a subluxation, causes nerve interference. Subluxations could cause breakdown or blockage in the body's communication network, which could lead to a wide range of health problems.

That's where chiropractors come in. We detect subluxations and correct them by performing specific adjustments. Adjustments to the spinal vertebrae release the natural healing properties God instilled in all of us. By receiving regular chiropractic adjustments, your child's body could be better equipped to defend against illness and injury.

Subluxations occur throughout our lives. Here are just a few that could occur in childhood:

- The birth process. Whether delivery is natural or surgical, birth places significant stress on babies' spines and nerves. The neck can be stretched during delivery, which can apply significant force. Thus, the first subluxation could occur quietly, often without detection.
- Development of basic motor functions in infancy such as holding up the head, crawling, walking and repeatedly falling.
- Spinal stress from heavy school backpacks.
- Sports injuries, from soccer to gymnastics.
- Emotional and social stresses of being a child in this world.
- Jungle gym and playground falls.
- Car accidents.

We have all experienced some of these causes of subluxation. The question is for how long, and to what severity, the subluxations have existed.

What are we doing to improve the health of our children? Are we making the best choices? Could children be medicated today, more than ever before? An abundance of medication options exist for children from antibiotics to behavior-modification drugs. Could some of these cover symptoms instead of helping us discover the cause of the problems?

Ear Infections

Consider Auriel, a 9-year-old who experienced repeated ear infections and hearing loss in her left ear. This young girl was prescribed dose after dose of antibiotics for three years, yet continued to see a reoccurrence of painful infections. Since the antibiotics did not work, her doctor performed surgery to insert a tube in her ear drum to allow for wax and fluid drainage.

Unfortunately, even the ear tube did not solve little Auriel's problem. The tubes did allow her ears to drain puddles of pungent, disgusting fluid on her pillow each night. But, the surgery failed to correct the cause of the problem. She was still plagued by frequent infections and communication difficulties.

Next, she lost her hearing in that ear, which affected Auriel's ability to learn and socialize in school. Struggling to hear clearly, Auriel began to read lips. Her grades began to drop. She became withdrawn in her classes.

This was the last straw for Auriel's parents, whose frustration had reached an all-time high. They brought her into my office for a check-up and were eagerly searching for answers.

Unfortunately, this is not an uncommon pediatric situation. During my completion of a Fellowship Degree in Chiropractic Pediatrics and Pregnancy, I learned valuable information about this difficult problem.

According to the 1993 *National Hospital Ambulatory Medical Care Survey*, the most frequent diagnosis for hospital emergency room visits was otitis media, better known as ear infections.

According to an Associated Press report sourcing the U.S. Public Health Service, "the condition (ear infections) leads between six million and eight million children to visit doctors' offices annually."

The article also explains the two most common forms of otitis media. This first is otitis media with effusion, (OME), which "has no symptoms other than fluid collection." The other, acute otitis media (AOM), which can have aches or fever and is "the ear infection that causes severe pain."

Dr. Alfred Berg, co-chair of a federal panel of experts and a professor at the University of Washington states in the article, "antibiotics, frequently used in the past, are of very limited value in treating the condition (OME). The panel concluded that antibiotics, at best, conferred only a 14 percent advantage over doing nothing. Antibiotics can cause side effects..."

OME can reduce hearing acuity at a time when children are learning to speak. For this reason, the condition has often been treated aggressively.

A study published in the *Journal of the American Medical Association* questioned the effectiveness of a common antibiotic, Amoxicillin, for treating chronic long-term ear infections where fluid builds in the middle ear and threatens speech development and hearing in children. This has prompted concern in parents and doctors.

This study reopened a scientific debate regarding a struggle for millions of children and their families: How should chronic ear infections, where fluid builds in the ear (OME), be treated in young children?

A *Journal of the American Medical Association* found amoxicillin "is not effective in the treatment of persistent asymptomatic middle ear ellusions (OME or fluid on the ear) in infants and children."

In my experience, the healing of ear infections could occur within a few weeks without drugs. Subluxations negatively affecting the health of the inner ear must be removed. These subluxations – typically in the neck and upper back – impede the nerve supply to the inner ear, which prevents normal drainage from the middle ear and lymphatic system. If fluid accumulates in the middle ear, it could become a breeding ground for viruses and bacteria.

In Auriel's case, after performing a thorough consultation and examination, I found severe subluxations in her upper neck. This affected the nerve supply to the ear and surrounding tissue. We began a course of gentle adjustments to her spinal column three times a week.

After the second week, the drainage from Auriel's ears stopped. After two months, her teachers noticed better awareness and her grades began to rise from C's and D's to B's and B-pluses. A follow-up hearing test indicated her hearing and speech had improved. Today, she's a happier, healthier child focused on school and play.

Silent subluxations caused during childhood could create problems which follow children into adulthood. Shouldn't we teach children, at a young age, the importance of preventative care for their bodies? We teach our children to eat right, grow spiritually and other key lessons. Why not teach them to be aware of their bodies' states of wellness?

First Checkup

Remember, the first subluxations could occur during birth. I believe the sooner the first checkup, the better. I adjusted my son, Luke, five minutes after he was born.

Adjustments can be performed gently and with very little force. An adjustment could be as gentle as the weight of your finger on the back of your hand.

Ongoing care need not be limited to times when children show symptoms. As a parent, strive to develop wellness within your family. By making your children aware of their health, one could head off serious medical problems in the future. Plus, a healthy body creates ideal conditions for a child to develop mentally and socially.

I feel the best way to launch your family wellness goal is a spinal checkup for adults and children. It is never too late to start a program of prevention. Seek a family-oriented chiropractor, one who is qualified to evaluate both adults and children.

As your child grows and develops, make periodic visits to the chiropractor to monitor growth, posture and development of his or her nervous system. Remember, most illnesses can be silent in the beginning and could grow for years before being noticed.

Choose to prevent health challenges before they become a problem. By utilizing chiropractic care you could create wellness for you and your family. By putting the focus on maintaining a healthy nervous system and spine, you and your children could reap the benefits of optimum health throughout your lifetimes.

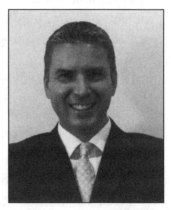

Dr. Craig T. French, D.C.
Chiropractic Pediatric Specialist
Chiropractic Professional Center
Monroeville, PA
412-372-5900
nervesrus@aol.com

PART FIVE

CHILDREN AND WELLNESS

⁂

By Dr. Jody A. Matthews, B.A., D.C.

The benefits of maintaining a healthy spine, from conception throughout life, could be astounding including immune system improvement, reduced need for medication and increased activity. A healthy spine, in my opinion, could allow a person to reach his or her fullest health potential.

Birth is a dynamic time to begin health and wellness. But no person is too old to experience an improved quality of life.

Providing the opportunity for a healthy life is my greatest desire. Seeing the results of chiropractic care is why I am passionate about what I do and excited to share with people how life can be changed forever!

Personal Belief

I suffered a football injury during college. Many unsuccessful attempts were made for recovery through traditional physical therapy and the orthopedic approach. I finally turned to a chiropractor for help.

Within two weeks of consistent adjustments, I was able to return to my college football career. My injury and recovery prompted my interest in becoming a chiropractor, so I could help other people.

During my second year of chiropractic care, I became aware

of the benefits beyond helping with my football injury when my lifelong battle with bronchitis ended. My immune system was the strongest it had ever been, confirming to me the power of a healthy spine and nervous system.

Chiropractic Today

Although I adjust patients of all ages, children are my greatest passion. Think of the newborn baby who experiences the trauma of birth. The natural birthing process could cause subluxation. This, in my opinion, left untreated could lower the baby's opportunity for optimal health and wellness.

The birthing process can be a beautiful experience without the need for drugs or pushing and pulling. My own son came into this world without drugs. From the minute he was born, he was alert and full of life.

Now at 20 months of age, he is still healthy and energetic. In fact, he has not missed one night of sleep from being ill.

In asking my new patients how many nights' sleep they have missed from taking care of sick babies, their responses are, "So many I can't count."

Tears still come to my eyes when I think back to the experiences my wife and I shared when our son was born. After learning about the potential risks associated with having our son immunized, my wife and I decided against it. Relaying this to our pediatrician, he immediately advised us that unless these immunizations were given, our son could become sick and die.

Preparing to leave the hospital, we were faced with a new challenge.

The hospital informed us that for our insurance company to cover the costs of our son's birth, a PKU test was required. Because this test only involved pricking the foot to obtain a blood sample and not injecting our son with medication, we allowed the test to be done when he was only 24 hours old.

However, after arriving at the pediatrician's office for follow up, we were told the PKU test performed at the hospital was invalid since it should have been performed when our son was more than 48 hours old.

Again, we heard the words, "without this test, your son could become sick and die." Can you imagine new parents being told their beautiful creation could die if a medical test were not performed?

My wife and I made the decision to stand our ground, refusing to have our son retested and what followed was a confirmation we made the right choice. The results from the PKU test were not available for six weeks and, of course, were negative.

If this test was invalid, why was an analysis of the test even performed? Secondly, if this test were a matter of life and death, why were the results not provided for six weeks? As parents, you have the power and the responsibility to question everything, demand answers and make independent decisions.

Spinal Correction at Birth

Another issue to address at birth is a chiropractic examination of the atlas bone, which is located where the spinal column and skull meet. Once this bone is aligned, I recommend it be checked three times within the first week. By the time your child reaches age one, a maintenance schedule consisting of monthly adjustments is recommended. From my own experience, I have seen my child's fever drop immediately after an atlas adjustment. I am not sure if this is from the change in the nervous system or relief to the nervous system but IT WORKED.

Immune System and Chiropractic

Dr. Edward Goetzl, M.D., professor of medicine and immunology at The University of California San Francisco, is lead author on a scientific paper published November 20, 2001 in *Proceedings of the National Academy of Sciences.*

The study confirmed the nervous system's direct influence on the immune system. Scientist found nervous system signals affect the migration of the immune system's T cells which is central to the body's normal defense against infection.

The most critical area of the nervous system is the brain stem. It is protected and surrounded by the atlas vertebrae. If the brain stem has even small interference from a misaligned or subluxated vertebra certain parts of the body could malfunction including the immune system.

Children and Chiropractic

Children are precious gifts. I believe, without proper chiropractic, they could suffer through many things they should never have to experience.

I often see parents with children who are suffering from earaches and other childhood sicknesses. One particular 12-month-old child had an ear infection so severe fluid was oozing from his ear. After adjusting this child, the ear cleared up and his sleeping habits improved dramatically.

You see, the body has an innate intelligence, a special inner wisdom. If a person has a minor cut, left alone, the cut will heal. Whether a person is five minutes or 95-years-old, properly aligned spines could allow the nervous system to clearly communicate with the body. Thus, the body could heal.

I am an ambassador for children's health and believe children should be given the ultimate opportunity in life.

One patient brought me her five-year-old son who was on four different types of asthma medication. Within the first week, he was off all the medications and now six months later he is 100% drug-free. The change was so remarkable, his mother received a letter from the boy's teacher stating he was no longer hyperactive in class and suggested the mother continue doing "whatever it was she was doing."

One of the major concerns regarding children is that they are given medication for everything, whether a headache, stomachache or common cold. If pain or illness is not gone within two days, the child is taken to the medical doctor who prescribes yet another pill.

Instead of rushing from one pill to another, the body, regardless of age, needs adequate time to heal.

What if you were the parent of a young girl whose spine was so out of alignment medical doctors diagnosed surgery to place a metal rod in your daughter's back? The doctors would likely tell you, with the surgery, your daughter's condition would not worsen, but they would not guarantee it would get any better. Would you automatically agree to the surgery because this is standard care? Or would you look for non evasive alternatives which could significantly help your child? Your decision will haunt or help your child for the rest of her life. With this surgery, your child's days of cheerleading, dancing and playing could come to an end.

Parents face a difficult challenge having to undo many years of believing in medical "crisis care." They may need to let go of their old philosophies for the sake of their children.

Health at Any Age

I have helped a woman break a 12-year dependency on antidepressants and regain optimal health and a renewed life. A 72-year-old patient of mine now enjoys optimal health because he has maintained chiropractic throughout his life.

Everyday people's lives are changed, immune systems are restored, activity levels are increased and quality of life is achieved. Although my passion is children, I care greatly about all my patients, regardless of age. My wish for everyone is to have a healthy spine so life can be experienced at its best!

Dr. Jody A. Matthews, B.A., D.C.
Lifetime Chiropractic, P.A.
Villa Rica, GA
770-459-5070
jchiroman@aol.com

PART SIX

IF YOU SLOUCH, YOU'RE GOING TO SAY, "OUCH, OUCH, OUCH!"

By Dr. Marvin Arnsdorff, D.C.

The Children's Spinal Wellness Movement

The children's spinal wellness movement is defined as the study of children (their physical characteristics, spinal health, posture and how they function) in relation to their activities of daily living (how they sit, stand, sleep, lift and carry objects such as backpacks). The goal of the children's spinal wellness movement is to prevent occurrence of future neuromusculoskeletal conditions such as neurological disorders, back and neck pain, repetitive stress injuries and more. By educating children in spinal health, proper "body mechanics" and healthy posture at an early age, we can help children grow up healthy with less pain. This could reduce the odds of future disability.

The True Posture Picture

Visit your local high school and count the number of kids who have dangerously poor posture. Take a poll of how many students are reporting back pain. You may find a number of children under the age of 18 reporting back pain. I believe this is steadily increasing. Another interesting insight would be to survey those with poor posture to determine how many are taking prescribed medications for an array of disorders from ADHD to asthma.

The Posture-Health Connection

It has been said, "Posture is the window to the spine." Therefore, wouldn't it make sense that if posture is misaligned, the spine inside is also misaligned? This could place unhealthy pressure on the spinal column and the nervous system.

Poor spinal health and posture can be seen as kids spend countless hours contorting themselves – improperly wearing their backpacks, sitting at computers, playing handheld computer games and watching television.

I believe posture is as important as eating right, exercising, getting a good night's sleep and avoiding harmful substances like alcohol, drugs and tobacco. Unnatural alignment of the body can cause head, shoulder, neck and back pain. It could also compromise neurological, digestive, respiratory and cardiovascular functioning.

Some adults with chronic spinal conditions could trace these problems to years of poor posture formed in early childhood. Most adults were never instructed as children on proper methods to sit, sleep, stand, lift and carry objects. And now, this lack of instruction causes industries, as required by the U.S. Occupational Safety and Health Administration (OSHA), to spend billions of dollars to impart knowledge. This education could have been delivered much less expensively and much more timely during childhood.

We have the need for a comprehensive children's spinal wellness movement. This is a preventive movement that would be supported by parents, educators and industry. Imagine the billions of dollars saved and the pain and suffering avoided if we empower children with a new model preventing future neuromusculoskeletal conditions from ever occurring.

The Look of Healthy Posture

Let's start by forgetting the benchmarks usually associated with having good posture. Except at charm school or West Point, balancing books on your head or standing rigidly at attention will not help the cause. Nagging children by saying, "Sit up straight," "Stand up straight" and "Stop slouching" is just as ineffective.

Children's spinal wellness includes the study of proper postural and ergonomic habits, regular spinal checkups (just like dental checkups) and exercises promoting spinal flexibility, strength and resiliency.

Consider the earlier statement, "Posture is the window to the spine." When posture is misaligned, then the spine inside is also affected. This can place unhealthy pressure on the spinal column and the nervous system. Thus, early detection and elimination of spinal imbalance (vertebral subluxation), through regular spinal checkups, could lead to a healthy spine and nervous system at each stage of a child's life.

The Four Steps of a Posture Check

Follow these simple steps to check a child's posture:

1. Standing behind the child, have the child close his or her eyes.
2. Check the level of the head, ears, shoulders and hips. If each is level, the spine is usually straight. If one side is higher than the other, a spinal curve may exist which could result in pressure on the joints, discs and nerves.
3. Now check from the side view. The ears should be directly over the shoulders. Shoulders should be directly over the hips. Hips should be directly over the knees. When this is not the case, there could be stress on the natural spinal curves.
4. If you see signs of posture imbalance or if your child has been complaining of neck, shoulder or back pain, you should have your child evaluated by a chiropractor.

Backpacks on the Attack

As a doctor of chiropractic, I have been alarmed by the number of children who, I feel, are improperly wearing backpacks and concerned about the repercussions to their health.

Guidelines for Proper Backpack Use

1. Choose Right – Choosing the correct size backpack is an important first step to safe backpack use. The backpack should not be larger than three quarters of the length of a child's back. The shoulder straps should be padded and a waist strap is ideal.
2. Pack Right – The maximum weight of the loaded backpack should not exceed 15% of your child's body weight, so only pack what is needed. The heavier books should be closer to the child. Regardless of the weight, if the backpack forces the wearer to bend forward to carry, it is overloaded.
3. Lift Right – Even adults can hurt themselves if they lift 20 pounds improperly. Imagine what a child could do to a growing spine by lifting 20 pounds improperly. Here are the guidelines for lifting a backpack:
   a) Face the pack
   b) Bend at the knees
   c) Use both hands and check the weight of the pack
   d) Lift with the legs
   e) Apply one shoulder strap, then the other
4. Wear Right – Use both shoulder straps snug, but not too tight (the pack should not hang down past the waist). When the backpack has a waist strap, it should be used.

Sitting Tall

We spend a large portion of our lives sitting, so let's make a point of teaching young ones how to sit properly early in life. One of the most common mistakes we make is while moving into a sitting position, we tend to aim for the center of the chair.

The proper method is to sit deep in your chair. While you sit, keep your shoulders back and your head over your shoulders.

Healthy Sleeping Positions

We sleep as much as a third of our lives, so proper positioning is critical to your health. I feel the first and most important idea is to not sleep on your stomach. If you sleep on your back, use one pillow to support your neck. A pillow under your knees will reduce pressure on your lower spine. If you sleep on your side, use a pillow to keep your head and neck level. When sleeping on your side, you can bend a bit at your hips and knees; don't curl up into a ball.

Posture for Healthy Computer Use

Students are spending more and more time at computers today. Here are nine simple guidelines designed for children using a computer at home or school:

1. Sit up straight and deep in the seat. Feet should be flat on the floor or on a footrest.
2. Keep lower arms level with the desk and wrists straight. (This can help prevent carpal tunnel syndrome.)
3. Sit close enough to your keyboard to eliminate stretching, but far enough to avoid leaning. Remember, your shoulders should be back and your head should be directly over your shoulders.
4. Tap the keyboard lightly; don't pound.
5. Place your mouse within easy reach of your dominant hand. Hold the mouse loosely.
6. Place the monitor at eye level and 16 to 24 inches away.
7. Take short stretch breaks every 20 minutes.
8. Exercise eyes frequently. Look away and focus on distant objects.
9. Periodically look up at the ceiling to give your posture muscles a break.

Lifting for Longevity

Proper lifting is important regardless of the size of what you're lifting (See the steps for proper lifting technique under backpacks). Remember, repetitive stress injuries occur over time. The accompanying pain can be the result of years of poor lifting habits. By lifting using the recommended steps in this chapter, you could help your children prevent years of painful existence.

Exercise and Stretching

To remain flexible and healthy for a lifetime, daily spinal and postural exercises are a must. Here's where you could see a major return on a minor investment of time. Ask your chiropractor for a recommendation on morning and evening routines requiring only a few minutes a day.

Prevent Now or Pay Later

Isn't it amazing that we take better preventative care of our teeth than our spine and nervous system? Get regular spinal checkups for you and your children!

Remember, good posture and body mechanics are an important part of having a healthy spine, nervous system and self-esteem.

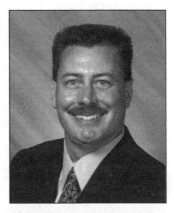

Dr. Marvin Arnsdorff, D.C.
Chiropractic USA
Mount Pleasant, SC
843-881-0046
www.bodymechanics.com
info@backpacksafe.com

Dr. Marvin Arnsdorff is a practicing doctor of chiropractic, a certified injury prevention specialist and leader of the children's spinal wellness movement. He is the author of *Pete the Posture Parrot™ Dinosaur Dreams*, the world's first children's book to address the issue of backpack safety, and co-author of *Backpack Safety America™: A Curriculum to Promote Backpack Safety and Spinal Health*.

PART SEVEN

A LIFETIME
OF WELLNESS

❧

By Dr. Colleen Trombley-VanHoogstraat, D.C. and
Dr. Marc VanHoogstraat, D.C.

Anyone who has witnessed the miracle of a baby developing in the womb followed by the birth of a bundle of joy must share in our awe at the perfect design of mothers and babies.

There are no diagrams or set of instructions for either. Our educated minds are forced to take a backseat to the wisdom of our innate intelligence. Left alone to unfold according to nature's grand design, and even with little outside assistance, all can be well with mother and child.

Many people have some form of spiritual "guidebook" to base their life decisions upon. For us, when it comes to the creation of optimal health and wellness, our guidebook is best exemplified by the principles of chiropractic.

The chiropractic principles are brilliant, yet simple. They are time-tested, rock-solid universal truths. Decisions regarding our family's health and future potential are effortless, consistent and congruent because we base them upon the infrastructure of this principled reasoning.

Recently, we were able to apply these beliefs to one of the most important endeavors in our lives…the creation of our first child! Wellness must begin when life itself begins.

We are born with a Divine intelligence, an inborn healer. We believe this intelligence is capable of creating perfect health and function for an entire lifetime.

The nervous system is the main highway of communication for this innate intelligence. We refer to the nervous system as the "master system" since it carries messages of life and intelligence to every cell and tissue of the body. It is the system on which all others depend for direction, guidance and balance.

When the nervous system is free of interference, flawless perfection could be the result. Interference to this flow of life is known as subluxation, which could rob us of our potential for optimal function, performance and life.

Subluxation is most commonly caused by subtle shifts in spinal vertebrae, resulting in distorted communication along the life line between the brain and body.

Doctors of chiropractic are health professionals trained in the detection and correction of subluxation. Chiropractic adjustments remove the blockage, restoring optimal flow of life and intelligence. This magical stream of life is what initiates the miracle of creation.

With this in mind, regular chiropractic check-ups can be the nucleus of prenatal care for families living wellness lifestyles. One of our first steps in the care of expectant families is to remind them this amazing process is under the direction of a much higher power... thank goodness!

A clear path along the mother's nervous system could allow the developing fetus to receive every ounce of intelligence it needs, as well as, keeping the mother as healthy as possible.

The powerful force directing this extraordinary sequence of events doesn't abandon us once we exit the womb. This innate intelligence remains with us during our lifetime surging along the nervous system.

True wellness depends upon the ongoing balance of mind, body and spirit beginning at the earliest time possible. A child can be checked for subluxation at birth to afford them the greatest opportunity for unobstructed life, optimal health and higher performances and functions. Chiropractic adjustments at this stage can be as gentle as a mother's caress, yet remove nerve interferences.

Birth trauma to the infant's cervical spine and cranium can result in headaches, inner ear problems, speech troubles, sight disturbances, respiratory disorders and other health challenges.

Chiropractic adjustments could be the most priceless gift to give a child.

Many parents are diligent in seeing their children receive routine well baby check-ups, yet often omit the crucial role of chiropractic wellness care. Chiropractic is not an alternative to medical treatment — the two balance each other.

Our definition of lifetime wellness is a balanced, proactive approach to health as opposed to a reactive response to symptoms and crises. Some people still have the misconception chiropractic is only about your back.

It is true, the mind and body are connected by the lifeline running through the spine. But chiropractic is so much more — it's really about your life. We like to describe what we do, as doctors of chiropractic, as protecting the integrity, strength and vitality of the bridge between the mind and body (the nervous system), allowing the whole person to express a lifetime of wellness.

Regardless of a person's age, condition or circumstance, many individuals could respond more effectively and appropriately to the world around them (mentally, emotionally, spiritually, physically and chemically) free of subluxations. The underlying premise of chiropractic is really so simple.

Chiropractic care can be a supportive, proactive means of creating a lifetime of vibrant, unlimited performance, health and wellness. Be all you can be by having yourself and your children checked for subluxation.

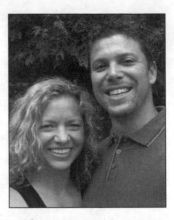

**Dr. Colleen Trombley-VanHoogstraat, D.C.
and Dr. Marc VanHoogstraat, D.C.**
Chiropractic USA
Oxford, MI
248-628-4886
powerzon@speedlink.net

Dr. Colleen Trombley-VanHoogstraat, D.C. and Dr. Marc VanHoogstraat, D.C. specialize in lifetime family wellness and peak performance.

CHAPTER FOUR

THE SCIENCE
OF SUBLUXATIONS

PART ONE

WHAT IS HEALTH?

❧

By Dr. Renny Edelson, D.C.

"What is health?"

This seemingly simple question leaves most people grasping for an accurate answer.

To enjoy a lifetime of wellness, it is important that every individual understand how to maintain the body in a healthy state.

Perhaps the easiest way to understand health is to first explore what health is not. For generations, our society has been raised to believe that "if it ain't broke, don't fix it."

In other words, until we begin showing symptoms of a problem, it is assumed we are healthy. This includes serious ailments such as heart disease and cancer, which seem to appear from nowhere.

But diseases do not simply materialize overnight. They could manifest themselves long before the first symptoms begin to appear.

The central nervous system, which is primarily comprised of the brain and spinal cord, is the central control system for the functions your body undertakes each day. For the central nervous system to function ideally, the spine must be free of decay and be properly aligned.

But the everyday stresses of life, plus occasional traumatic episodes, cause people to have misalignments of the spine called subluxations. These misalignments could create devastating pressure and stress on the nervous system, decreasing the body's overall wellness.

Surprisingly, about 90 percent of subluxations are silent. They initially cause no symptoms as the body fights to cope with them. By the time signs of a problem appear, serious damage may have already been done.

If you are experiencing a sign of illness, a prescription might be written for you. By choosing this approach, you may experience relief from symptoms. But, the underlying illness could remain untreated.

Could our bodies be naturally designed to heal?

Chiropractic could help create optimal healing by removing interferences to your body's own natural abilities to heal.

Rather than treating individual symptoms, we view health from a holistic standpoint. Chiropractors look at health from the inside out. We appreciate the body's ability to heal.

Some people think that age affects healing ability. Once they pass 30-, 50- or 80-years-old, their bodies lose ability to heal. Not so. Whether you are eight or 80-years-old, if you cut yourself, the body will heal that cut. Broken bones may have to be set, but they mend on their own over time.

When God created mankind, He was not so tricky as to hide away the secrets to health and healing. He didn't create a treasure hunt for wellness. I believe He placed the power to heal within each and every one of us.

To unlock this powerful healing mechanism, you could begin by ensuring your spinal health. Make a decision to have your spinal alignment checked regularly throughout life starting as early as birth.

Remember, the state of your spinal health changes over time. Stress takes its toll, whether physical, emotional or chemical. Stress could put pressure on your spine, causing misalignments that could lead to health problems later in life.

Removing this pressure is like straightening out a bend in a garden hose. It restores the flow of energy and information, enabling the body to increase its healing powers.

I know of high-profile sports figures choosing to maintain optimum health through spinal adjustments. For example, Tiger Woods and Lance Armstrong have personal chiropractors who regularly check their spinal health. Top-performing athletes, like these, function at the highest capacity possible, in part, by taking care of their spines.

But this care is not limited to the high-profile athletes. Preventative chiropractic care is an affordable option for everybody in our society.

To illustrate the profound effect of spinal health on overall wellness, consider the study authored by Dr. Henry Windsor, M.D and published in *The Medical Times*.

In 1921, this groundbreaking researcher questioned the effectiveness of chiropractic care. He doubted the theory that misalignments of the spine caused diseases in other parts of the body.

At the University of Pennsylvania, Dr. Windsor dissected 75 human cadavers during two studies to investigate their causes of death.

He traced the nerves from "sick" organs to their origins on the spinal column. Dr. Windsor found 139 diseases in the first study of 50 cadavers such as 15 bodies with lung pneumonia, 5 with gallstones, 4 with bronchitis, 1 with larynx cancer, 11 with cirrhosis, 4 with enlarged prostate gland, 7 with enlarged spleen and 15 with enlarged kidneys.

In 138 of the 139 diseases, Dr. Windsor found a correlation between "minor curvatures" of the vertebrae and diseases of internal organs. This included cases of disease in organs such as the heart, lungs, liver, throat, pancreas, gallbladder, stomach, spleen, kidney, uterus, prostate and bladder. In each of the 138 cases, misalignments (subluxations) occurred in the spine where the nerves were located and began travel to these diseased organs.

Even more profound was Dr. Windsor's conclusion, "The organs were in many instances affected by acute disease, while the deformed vertebrae proved that the curvatures (spinal misalignments) preceded the organic diseases..."

What better example of the importance of spinal health?

I believe that everyone wants to be healthy. Nobody wants to grow old and have oatmeal dripping from their chin in a nursing home while they wait for their family to visit.

Remember, health is not about what you feel. With only about 10 percent of your body's nerves dedicated to feeling pain, your internal systems could be malfunctioning long before you feel discomfort. Living life as though you are healthy, simply because you have few to no symptoms, is not an acceptable path to health.

By embracing spinal checkups and adjustments when necessary, you could benefit from better overall health. Could this equate to less medication? And, according to Dr. Windsor's research, chiropractic patients could avoid developing chronic illnesses requiring ongoing medication.

Protect your precious health. Don't wait for the pain to take action. Don't wait for a frightening diagnosis of serious illness. Make regular deposits in your health account, and you will be blessed with wealth that comes from wellness.

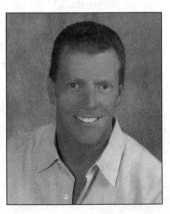

Dr. Renny Edelson, D.C.
Chiropractic USA
Plantation, FL
954-581-1999

PART TWO

ARE YOU HEALTHY?

By Dr. Becky Simmons, D.C. and Dr. Greg Ramboer, D.C.

Wellness is experienced when you are at your absolute best...mentally, physically, emotionally and spiritually. This could be a lifelong journey of restoring and maintaining health.

It's possible a patient may need to make a structural spinal correction before his or her body is in a state conducive to wellness. Proper structure of the spine and nervous system could lead to optimal function and optimal health. Proper spinal alignment allows nerve messages from the brain to the body, ultimately life itself, to flow freely with no interruption. Like a fine instrument, the body performs best when perfectly tuned.

Health and wellness are not merely the absence of disease, but also the presence of optimal function. In a state of wellness, the body functions at its absolute highest potential.

We believe it is a universal principle that the human body has an amazing, flawless ability to adapt and to heal itself using its own innate or inborn intelligence. When a health problem is evident, it could be because the body's powerful healing abilities have been inhibited.

We feel there is a major difference between managing a health problem and maintaining health. If a person in pain takes a pill and the pain goes away, does this mean he or she is healthy again?

A headache could commonly be associated with an improper

cervical curve in the neck. Taking a pill may cover up the symptom, but the root cause (the improper curve) could still exist. This could cause the headache symptom to return. Is it possible, in chiropractic, if a patient only comes in when headaches occur, then stops care until the pain returns that he or she might simply be managing the problem?

We believe it could be nearly impossible to exhibit total wellness in a situation like this. We call this crisis care, not health (or wellness) care.

The goal of wellnesscare is to restore and maintain health by correcting the source of health problems, not just the pains. Wellnesscare could consist of weekly, biweekly or monthly chiropractic check-ups, determined by individual response. Until they begin regular chiropractic care, many people don't realize it's possible to increase how well they feel.

"If I Feel Well, I Must Be Healthy?"

Even though a person feels well, or doesn't have symptoms, it doesn't mean his or her body is functioning at 100 percent. Damaging nerve interference could be present and unknown. This silent interference, or subluxation, could choke the full expression of life in our bodies. Seek the professional abilities of a chiropractor to check for and remove subluxation.

The earlier subluxation is detected and corrected, the better a person's chance is to perform at her or his highest potential. We prefer to start spinal adjustments at the earliest age possible.

Birth could be one of the most traumatic processes in a person's life. A tremendous amount of pressure and stress is put on the spinal cord when the baby is being pulled and twisted through the birth canal. It can be a major cause of subluxation for the mother and child.

As reported by the Children's Chiropractic Research Foundation, birth trauma to the cervical spine and cranium can result in the following in infants:

- headaches,
- vestibular problems (inner ear),
- auditory troubles (speech),
- visual disturbances (sight),
- pharyngolaryngeal disorders (the canal between mouth and esophagus),
- vasomotor dysfunction (relating to the nerves and muscles causing blood vessels to constrict or dilate) and
- secretion dysfunction

We believe a compromised nervous system causes ill health. Spinal check-ups promote optimal physical, emotional and intellectual development bringing children back toward wellness. The spine is both the backbone of the human body and the backbone of good health.

If the cause of ill-health is removed, doesn't it make sense your inner innate wisdom could heal the body? Chiropractic care could reveal a whole new, better you!

Results of a wellness and quality of life study of 2,818 chiropractic patients, conducted by University of California College of Medicine Professor Dr. Robert H.L. Blanks, Ph.D., indicted that chiropractic patients reported significant, positive enhancements in their physical health, abilities to deal with mental and emotional stress and increase in overall confidence, well-being and enjoyment of life.

Findings from the same survey indicated 99% of the chiropractic patients said they were choosing to continue chiropractic care even though a majority (96%) rated themselves in good to excellent health.

Four Essentials

Take a moment to consider the four essentials of life: Food, water, air and nerve supply. The average person could live without food for about 30 to 50 days. He or she could survive a few days without water. Without air, the brain could die within minutes. However, if you cut the nerve supply from the brain to the spinal cord, the person would die near instantaneously.

This is a simple scientific fact. Your nervous system controls everything. Nerve impulses flowing from the brain through the spinal cord and out to the body are the most essential part of life.

You can eat the healthiest foods on the planet, but it doesn't matter if there is nerve interference to the stomach not allowing proper digestion.

What are you doing to improve the quality of your nervous system? No one else can be responsible for your health and the health of your family. Choose to take control and be proactive. Being proactive might require a healthier diet, more exercise, stress management, proper rest, a positive attitude and, most importantly, spinal health check-ups by a chiropractor on a regular basis.

The greatest gift you can give your loved ones is a complete spinal evaluation by a doctor of chiropractic. Chiropractic is about living a higher quality of life and should be the first choice on a path toward wellness. Be the best you can be!

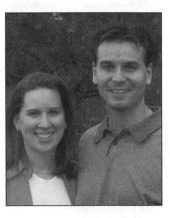

Dr. Becky Simmons, D.C.
Dr. Gregory Ramboer, D.C.
Lifepointe Chiropractic Center
Clarkston, MI
248-623-6107

Dr. Gregory Ramboer and Dr. Becky Simmons are chiropractic doctors who are dedicating their lives to enhancing the health of others. They specialize in family wellness and practice at Lifepointe Chiropractic Center in Clarkston, Michigan 248-623-6107.

PART THREE

OPTIMAL SPINE =
OPTIMAL HEALTH

❧

By Dr. Mark J. Casertano, D.C., BS, ATC, NMT

Normal spinal structure, attainable through chiropractic care, is essential for sound nerve function and optimal health.

When subluxations are corrected, proper communication is then restored from the brain to the body via the nervous system. Spinal subluxations can be corrected and rehabilitated. In addition, changes must be made in the osseous structure, muscles and ligaments. This correction involves a three-step process.

Three Step Process

First, the *nervous system* is directly affected by performing the chiropractic adjustment. Second, the *muscles* are affected by posture exercises. Third, the *ligaments* are reeducated using various types of therapeutic traction.

1. **Nervous System** – Once the nervous system has been subjected to stress due to subluxation, proper communication to the organs and muscles can be affected. In my opinion, when given the right opportunity, the body can perform miracles. When the body is in a crisis, after interference is eliminated, it has an amazing healing power.

2. **Muscle** – Performing chiropractic adjustments to the spine may slowly remove scar tissue. This could allow for an increased range of motion in the joints and removal of mi-

nor displacements of the bone rejuvenating optimal nerve flow. Performing specific exercises for soft tissue components can be an essential tool for patients to reach optimal health. Unless the muscles and ligaments are addressed, any change achieved might only be temporary.

3. **Ligaments** – Left in a state of subluxation, the body can only accommodate a crisis for so long before something serious occurs. Patients must take responsibility for their own health by modifying their daily activities that may be a contributing factor to their subluxation pattern. Achieving optimal results is a team effort between both patient and doctor.

Regular spinal checkups are necessary to minimize the possibility of undetected subluxation. Just as having your teeth cleaned regularly promotes healthy teeth, the spine also requires maintenance to maintain proper alignment. For example, think of a person with poor dietary habits. Although this person may have a higher risk of fatal heart attack from clogged arteries, the actual blockage cannot be felt. Subluxation is similar. It cannot be felt, although the results can manifest in many ways.

Nine-Year-Old Patient

My practice includes patients that suffer from various disorders. One particular patient was a nine-year-old female, living with a spinal disorder caused by the absence of a specific gene within chromosome five. The result is damage to the part of the spinal cord controlling motor function. As the disease progresses, the muscles continually weaken and affect life-sustaining organs, ultimately stopping the heart from beating and the lungs from expanding.

Prior to my care, this patient underwent extensive tests confirming the severity of her disease, which according to her medical doctors meant that nothing could be done.

Upon my examination, she presented severe weakness in all

her limbs due to atrophy of the muscles, severely decreased range of motion in all joints, severe thoracic scoliosis complicating her breathing, head in flexion (chin to chest) and legs bent in a 90-degree angle from spending life in a wheelchair.

The process of rehabilitation began. Within a few visits, she regained 50% mobility. This resulted in an improved ability to hold her head upright. After seven months of being under consistent care, she became stronger, sat upright and experienced an increased quality of life.

Upon returning to the hospital for a routine checkup, the specialists were excited by the improvements made since her last visit. Her doctors questioned me and her father regarding what type of care had been given. The chiropractic adjustments were explained. The doctors responded saying she had made great improvements, and I should continue doing what I was doing.

This special little girl is on the road to reaching her full expression and wish of achieving optimal health.

Cases such as this are what keep me and other chiropractors excited about what we do. Giving hope to people who have exhausted all other avenues for overcoming sickness, malfunction and injury is my mission. I do this by helping people achieve and maintain proper spinal structure.

Personal Experience

I believe in and am passionate about what I do both from patients' results and my personal experience.

I have been actively involved with sports throughout my life. At an early age, I realized the importance of chiropractic care through regular visits to our family chiropractor. I could tell these visits minimized my incidences of illness and injury.

One Injury Above the Rest

It was an injury suffered while playing football in high school, resulting in a dislocated shoulder. My mother took me directly from the game to the family chiropractor. Within six days, I was back on the field unlike a fellow teammate who suffered the same injury. He was taken to the hospital and placed in a sling for four weeks. What makes chiropractic care so powerful is it enables the body to become an amazing healing machine.

Today, I maintain my health and apply it to everything I do in life. I have competed and won many bodybuilding titles while in Georgia and New York State. Chiropractic care is one of the key elements, along with passion, commitment, diet and exercise, in attaining and maintaining my body's optimal performance. My goal is to see chiropractic care become incorporated into every family's lifestyle.

Chiropractic care has been stereotyped solely as neck and back pain relief for far too long. Each person in the family, including newborns, should be checked for subluxations. Most people do not realize during the birthing process subluxations can occur in both the mother and child. In my opinion, chiropractic care results in productive and healthy lives.

I believe wellness to be the balanced interaction between mind, body, and spirit. The benefits may include enhanced immune function, vitality and increased mental acuity. The result can be optimal health. This is what I am dedicated to and I would encourage everyone to seek chiropractic care and experience its many life-changing benefits.

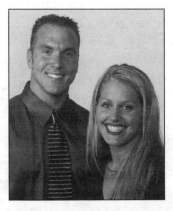

Dr. Mark J. Casertano, D.C., BS, ATC, NMT
Dawn M. Casertano
Chiropractic and Sports Injury
of North Fulton
Alpharetta, GA
770-740-1255

PART FOUR

WINNING THE GAME
OF HEALTH

✦

By Dr. Thomas E. Grant Jr., D.C.

It is 1st and goal, your football team is set to score. The messenger, with details on the winning play, runs to your huddle from the sideline bench. To your shock, out of nowhere, the opposing team tackles your messenger before he makes it to your huddle.

You shout for a penalty, but the play clock has started. You are forced to run a quick, uncoordinated play.

It's 2nd down. You can hardly believe what just happened. The play messenger comes out toward your huddle with the next play. He gets creamed again! "This is crazy," you think. "Why aren't the referees calling a penalty against the other team?"

The 3rd down comes. Again, no player from your bench can even get close to you with the coach's winning play.

Suddenly, you realize you've lost the ball and a chance to win the game. "Not fair," you shout, but it happened anyway.

What if this is what happened to you with every play in every game? Could you have the energy or desire to play the game for long? Would you ever win?

This is what could happen every moment of every day when your spinal nerves are blocked by vertebral subluxation.

Subluxation is like the opposing football team who won't let your play messenger get out to your huddle. Subluxation doesn't allow messages to get through your nervous system. Subluxation's job is to knock out the messenger before the message from your coach (your brain) gets to your body for the right function to occur.

To provide the best protection for your nerve system, you need a great defense. A subluxation free spine, which is maintained with correct spinal posture, is your most powerful protection.

What is Correct Spinal Posture?

Your spinal alignment is commonly referred to as your "posture." Whether short or tall, small or large, young or old, each of us has a certain posture. We each have a way of living that may influence how our spine grows.

The way you sit, stand, sleep, run, jump and play could all have effects on the structure of your spine. This, in turn, could directly influence the way your body functions. I believe, to maximize your health, you must understand how the shape and motion of your spine affects the function of your body.

When a baby is born, two of its four natural spinal curves are already in place at the torso and tailbone. After birth, a baby begins development of the other two normal curves of the spine at the neck and low back. These natural curves are C-shaped at the neck and an ellipse shape at the low back. Over time, however, the shape of those curves may be altered by gravity, life traumas and sometimes disease. The pain and discomfort of poor posture could curtail or even halt the activities of our daily living.

From the moment of conception, your developing body has innate knowledge of how to form your spinal cord into a perfect spine.

If that perfectly designed spine is not achieved or becomes altered, the spinal cord may not adapt well to the new shape. When certain spinal stresses occur, a wide variety of problems could result.

What does poor posture feel like? There could be many symptoms expressed by a poorly aligned spine. What is the condition of your spine? Assess your body's comfort level. Are you experiencing any of these symptoms?

- tightness in your neck or shoulders
- head jutting forward
- headaches
- tightness in the lower back
- aching calves
- feelings of stress or fatigue
- stiffness or reduced flexibility

If you are bothered by any of these issues, you might have a problem with your posture. Chiropractic care could be your answer. Make an appointment with a chiropractic doctor to have your posture and symptoms evaluated.

How Do You Correct Poor Posture?

A chiropractor can determine the possible causes of improper posture by utilizing diagnostic testing. These tests may include posture evaluation, an x-ray examination and a detailed analysis of your spinal curvature. During this evaluation, your chiropractor may find subluxations, or misalignments, of your spine.

If subluxations exist, the chiropractic doctor will usually begin a course of adjustments. This may be followed by spinal curve corrective care using specialized stretches, exercise or traction. This can help to relieve unwanted pressure on your nerves, realign your spine, improve your posture and help restore your health.

Spinal adjustments are performed in my office on a specialized adjusting table that assists in subluxation correction and posture training. These adjustments help restore integrity to the spine.

In my opinion, life-long wellness requires healthy posture. For longer-lasting results, I recommend my patients adopt lifestyle behavioral changes that support spinal corrections. Unfortunately, some people have developed poor posture habits. Innocently enough, these poor posture habits could actually harm health.

To create good posture and protect the spine, new habits may need to be developed. I teach patients what I believe to be the proper way to sit, stand erect and relax the body.

Stretching to Good Health

After initiating spinal adjustments, I start my patients on the second phase of their care: a course of individualized traction and stretching. This is non-surgical, painless care specifically designed for correcting posture.

When muscles are tight, over time, the ligaments surrounding the bones of the spine could gradually shorten. This could limit flexibility. By using specialized traction care, we can naturally stretch ligaments. The goal of this care is better flexibility and improved posture.

To be completely effective in reaching our care goals, stretching must continue at home. I recommend several that continue to tone and stretch the muscles and ligaments. These stretches help relieve stress in the shoulders, neck and the full spine.

Empowering each person to take charge of his or her own health is a high priority for me.

The next essential step to posture correction, in my opinion, is exercise. The ligaments are lengthening. They require strong muscles to support their new state of health. A program of individualized exercise strengthens the muscles and supports healthy spinal posture. These exercises could also help patients increase motion and flexibility.

Motion, or the ability to move, is necessary for a vibrant, fulfilling life. As we lose motion in our spine, the body stiffens.

Certain body functions may start slowing down. This lack of function could lead to premature aging or even untimely death.

Walking, playing and other physical activities bring flexibility to spinal joints and discs. Physical activities can increase blood supply to the spine. Without physical activity, the joints and discs could deteriorate and lead to compromised health.

Improved spinal structure could create several benefits. The body could be strengthened. The spine and nervous system pressure could drop considerably. Posture improvements could have you looking and feeling better and more youthful. The body may be able to accelerate the healing process, adapting and improving its state of health.

Is poor posture and loss of flexibility stealing your life away? Do you know someone who has lost their ability to live produc tively?

Spinal adjustments could improve your health. Why not make a commitment to your good health by participating in a holistic program of chiropractic care? This life-enhancing regiment could help you reach your goals of health and wellness, including restoration of the body's strength and power.

Empower your life through improved posture. Better health and a better world could be your re- ward. Allow a chiropractor to coach you to reach your goal of winning the game of health.

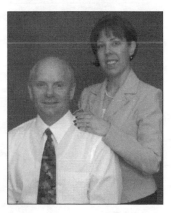

Dr. Thomas E. Grant Jr., D.C.
Kimberli Grant, ACRRT
Grant Chiropractic, LLC
Fayetteville, GA
770-719-1917
www.grantchiropractic.com

Dr. Thomas Grant Jr. is the inventor of the Adjust Pro™ Table and Align-a-Spine™. Dr. Grant specializes in chiropractic biophysics.

PART FIVE

Disease Caused by Nerve Interference

By Dr. Shane Hand, D.C.

"Get knowledge of the spine, for this is the requisite of many diseases." – Hippocrates

My practice is based on helping my patients find health and wellness by reducing and eliminating subluxations or misalignments of the spine. Your spine's alignment actually determines how well energy flows from your brain through your spine and on to your vital organs and muscles. This is called nerve flow.

Nerve flow could affect how well your immune system works. I believe God designed your body to be healthy. With proper nerve flow, your immune system could defend against all sorts of diseases. When nerve flow is slowed or blocked because of subluxation, your immune system could become compromised.

Pain, sickness and untimely death could result from subluxation because nerve flow is an important factor in our state of health. Through chiropractic adjustments, subluxations could be reduced or even eliminated, restoring nerve flow. As a result, true health and wellness could be restored.

I begin an appointment with both an x-ray and a computerized analysis of my patients' spines. The x-ray gives us a visual picture of the curves in the neck and spine, as well as, helping pinpoint any misalignments. Sometimes the misalignments are subtle; and sometimes they are truly obvious, reflecting years of twisting and distortion.

The computerized analysis includes electromyography, which is a way to detect nerve interference. Electromyography is used to measure the amount of electrical activity within muscle fibers. A reduced electrical activity could be a sign of subluxation. These tools help me determine care and educate each patient. They also allow patients to see the progress we are making.

Cause of Subluxation

Vertebral subluxation could be due to unaddressed or cumulative:

• Physical Stress
• Chemical Stress
• Emotional stress

Examples of physical stress could be trauma, injury or repetitive tasks. Chemical stress could be related to the use of drugs, poor diet and pollution. Emotional stress could deal with your job, family and social issues. Emotional stressors can be difficult to change quickly, therefore emotional stress ranks high.

When people are asked about why they seek chiropractic treatment, the most common answer is due to injury or trauma. Chiropractic was not intended to be solely a treatment for pain. It is for the detection and correction of subluxation.

Although many, if not most, people try chiropractic because of physical trauma, properly educated, they begin to see the whole picture. They start to address the emotional and chemical stresses in their lives. It's amazing what chiropractic care can actually accomplish in terms of restoring compromised health.

In 2001, Debra came to me looking for relief from some of her symptoms. She had been on dialysis three times a week for six years because her kidneys had failed and atrophied. She also had a kidney transplant in 1993 and after two months that kidney failed. When she arrived she was badly bloated and feeling sick most of the time. Her examination revealed severe subluxation in the lumbar region, her spine and nerves badly twisted. The nerves from the lumbar spine supply the kidneys with the power to function properly.

After a few adjustments, she began to feel better and decided to continue working with me while she waited for a kidney transplant. In her own words, she said, "After about three or four months of going two to three times or more a week, I began making some urine for the first time in one-and-a-half to two years."

Debra isn't cured by any means. The damage to her kidneys is severe enough to still require a transplant. She is much stronger and less bloated. The atrophied kidneys are actually beginning to function.

She is currently on the list for another kidney. I believe, this time, her chance for success with a new kidney is much better. By gradually reducing the subluxation of her spine and improving her nerve flow, I believe we turned on her God given innate power to heal. This is just one example of how nerve flow affects the body's major organs.

Children Benefit Too!

Chiropractic care isn't limited to adults. Children often benefit as well. One of my patients, Elise, was only 14-years-old on her first visit. Even at such a young age, she had been suffering severe headaches and migraines for years.

The pain was so severe Elise was unable to attend school regularly for four years. Several doctors including two neurologists, an allergist, a cardiologist, a rheumatologist, a physiatrist and an ear, nose and throat specialist had attempted to relieve Elise's migraines with little or no success.

My analysis revealed Elise had many subluxations in her neck area. I believe these could have been caused during birth, especially if the birth attendant turned Elise's head, up to 90 degrees, to facilitate passage through the birth canal.

Chiropractic adjustments relieved Elise's severe headaches. She is no longer suffering migraines. One of the most interesting facts about this case is Elise is a twin; and her twin didn't suffer migraines or headaches.

Health Care Options

The chiropractic method is a natural approach to health, healing and wellness.

It's interesting the *Journal of the American Medical Association* (*JAMA*) published a commentary by Dr. Barbara Starfield, MD, on July 26, 2000 which stated the third leading cause of death behind heart disease (750,000 deaths per year), and cancer (500,000 deaths per year) is iatrogenic deaths totaling approximately 225,000 deaths per year.

According to *Webster's College Dictionary*, iatrogenic death means "induced unintentionally by the medical treatment of a physician."

The iatrogenic death total includes 12,000 deaths per year from unnecessary surgery, 7,000 deaths per year from medication errors in hospitals, 20,000 deaths per year from other errors in hospitals, 80,000 deaths per year from nosocomial infections in hospitals and 106,000 deaths per year from adverse effects of medications.

According to *Webster's College Dictionary*, nosocomial infections are "infections contracted in a hospital."

This total is for deaths only and does not include adverse effects associated with disability or discomfort.

Chiropractic Care

Chiropractic emphasizes proper nerve system function through adjustments, good posture, diet and exercise.

An integral part of my practice is encouraging my patients

to have their children checked for subluxlations. The spine should be maintained from birth to prevent problems and crisis down the road. When you understand the nerve system is your body's master system, it makes sense to get it checked for optimal performance especially at a young age.

I truly believe chiropractic adjustments can save lives. My chiropractic practice allows me to truly make a positive difference.

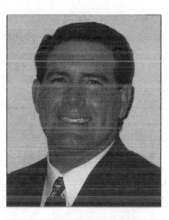

Dr. Shane Hand, D.C.
Hand Family Chiropractic
Amarillo, TX
806-373-4263

PART SIX

THE WINDOW
TO WELLNESS

༄

By Dr. Charles T. Francis, D.C.

"Stand up straight!"

How many times did you hear those words from your parents? Well, it turns out they were right. Your posture has a significant impact on your health and quality of life.

If you did not know about the strong link between posture and wellness, you're not alone. Even some physicians do not understand the importance of good posture, other than the fact better posture looks more pleasing to the eye.

So how can posture affect the body? Simple. Your posture is a direct representation of your spine, and therefore your health. If your posture is abnormal, chances are the structure of your spine is abnormal as well.

The central nervous system is composed of the brain and spinal cord, which control every physiological function in our bodies. So if the spine is abnormal, it could place dangerous stress and pressure on the central nervous system. This pressure on the spinal cord affects the brain's ability to communicate with the rest of the body.

To know whether your spine and central nervous system are healthy, you must determine whether your posture is normal. A chiropractor can do this for you. Here is a simple "self test" you can use prior to seeing a chiropractor. This test, however, is not meant to replace the advice or diagnosis of a doctor of chiropractic.

To evaluate your posture accurately, you must check it from both the front and the side.

Start with your body directly in front of a full length mirror. Close your eyes and march in place to loosen up the body. Then, with your eyes remaining closed, stand as straight as you possibly can. At this point, your body thinks it is displaying correct posture.

Now open your eyes and evaluate what you see. Starting from the space directly between your ankles, imagine a vertical line rising straight up from the floor. If you have normal posture, that line should pass through points in the center of your pubic bone, through your navel, between your collar bones, through your chin and between your eyebrows. Also, your shoulders and hips should be level with one another, and your head should not tilt or rotate to either side.

To evaluate your posture from the side, you will need a friend's help. As before, close your eyes and march in place. Then stand as straight as possible. This time, the starting point is the side of your ankle. An imaginary vertical line should rise upward and pass through the side of your knee, the side of your hip, the center of your shoulder joint and the center of your ear hole. If any point falls outside of the line, it could indicate there is a spinal misalignment.

The most common misalignment seen is the head jutting forward from the body when looking at the side view. A head excessively forward could be the result of trauma, such as a car accident. But, just as often, this condition develops from our lifestyle including hours at a computer, a long amount of time behind the wheel of a car or sleeping on a mound of pillows.

This condition could lead to neck and spinal problems causing symptoms such as headaches, dizziness, soreness in the neck and upper back and burning, numbness or tingling in the extremities.

If your posture is abnormal, yet you feel no pain, do not assume that you are problem-free. Just as a cavity can eat into your tooth long before you develop a toothache, so could other health problems develop without your awareness of pain. Only approximately 10 percent of the body's nerves are dedicated to pain sensation, with the other 90 percent controlling body function. Poor posture could lead to pain, spinal degeneration (arthritis) and deteriorating health. Your posture could show you something is wrong, long before the discomfort starts.

Picture the tires on your car. If they are not balanced properly, they tend to wear in certain spots. Just as the longevity of a car's tires can be protected by proper alignment, so can your body.

A healthy posture and healthy spine depend upon chiropractic care as a solid foundation. They also require two other major elements: good spinal hygiene and proper spinal alignment.

What is Spinal Hygiene?

Spinal hygiene is the maintenance and well-being of your spine from birth. Unlike dental hygiene, we are not taught to take daily care of and maintain the health of our spine. That is why a number of people can develop spinal problems during their lifetime.

Good spinal hygiene starts with a simple awareness of how we sit and stand. According to a 1970 study by Nachemson and Elfstrom, when the body stands, it bears 100 percent of its weight. When lying down, it bears less than 100 percent. But when sitting, the lumbar discs can bear an astonishing 200 percent of the body's weight.

Normal, healthy spines can bear the additional pressure of sitting comfortably without any symptoms. However, if you have a spinal misalignment and/or loss of the normal spinal curvatures, sitting could easily compound problems in an already compromised area. That is why I have come to the conclusion that people with an undiagnosed and untreated spinal misalignment have difficulty driving or sitting for any period of time.

If you work sitting at a desk most of the day, try to incorporate standing into your routine. Also, make sure the computer screen is eye-level. You should be looking directly at the middle of the screen as you work, which will take additional stress off of your neck and shoulders.

The chair you sit in should support your back comfortably. Avoid slouching or sitting in chairs that do not provide low back support, which will further increase the pressure to your spine.

Subluxations from Sleeping

At night, refrain from sleeping on your stomach. This position causes many spinal problems. It forces you to turn your head to one side or the other, twisting your neck and applying torque to the spine. Pillows compound this problem, raising your neck up higher and bending your neck sideways. When sleeping on your back with stacked pillows, your neck is pushed in an unnatural forward position. This could result in spinal misalignment and potentially close down the airway, which can cause snoring.

The two ways I recommend people sleep are either on your back, with no pillows or a small roll under your neck, or on your side. When sleeping on your side, the pillow needs to be high enough to keep your head, neck and face parallel to the bed. Postural positioning while sleeping is important because sleep comprises more than 25 percent of your lifetime.

Spinal Alignment

The second element of postural and spinal health is spinal alignment. Spinal alignment can be self-checked with the easy and accurate postural assessment outlined earlier in this chapter. I would always recommend the professional diagnosis of a doctor of chiropractic.

Your chiropractor can determine the longevity, severity and correction of the spinal misalignments. Spinal misalignments, also known as subluxations, can be addressed properly by a chiropractor. Chiropractors are the health care professionals trained to detect and correct subluxations.

By getting to the root of your poor posture today, you could tune up your central nervous system and add years of great health to your life.

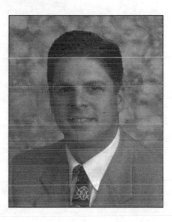

Dr. Charles T. Francis, D.C.
Francis Chiropractic
Charlotte, NC
704-759-9020
dr.francis@francischiropractic.com
www.francischiropractic.com

PART SEVEN

WELLNESS FOR LIFE

❧

By Dr. Robert C. Dees, D.C., RT

For 13 years, I have provided chiropractic care, currently in San Ramon, California. My passion is working with patients and educating them on the importance of a healthy spine. My name is Dr. Robert Dees and I want to provide people with valuable information on achieving "Wellness for Life."

Over time, a wide swing in the pendulum has occurred regarding healthcare. Do you know people who are tired of drugs that only mask the pain, tired of surgery and eager for natural alternatives?

Think about the traditional medical care you have received. In your experience, has this care focused more on treating pain and symptoms or the cause of your body's malfunction?

Valuable Care

Both medical doctors and chiropractic doctors have valuable places in society.

Medical doctors play an important role when it comes to "crisis care."

The chiropractors' expertise revolves around preventative wellnesscare and education.

The differences I see are medical doctors have a philosophy of health coming from outside-the-body-in. Chiltpractic doctors believe health comes from the inside-the-body-out.

Teaching Health and Wellness

I teach my patients that wellness is not related to a lack of pain, but to the nervous system perfectly communicating with every organ, muscle and tissue within the body.

I first began seeing patients on a symptomatic basis. I quickly discovered the immense importance of maintenance. I changed my philosophy from focusing on the patients' symptoms to teaching them new ways of life and wellness through chiropractic care.

The Subluxation Lesson

Subluxation is a serious condition where spinal bones are not properly aligned. Misalignment could result in nerve interference directly influencing body functions and healing.

Exercise, stress-free living, healthy diets, supplements and consistent chiropractic care are all valuable tools for achieving and maintaining a healthy lifestyle.

When patients tell me they have seen a chiropractor before but had no improvement, my response is to ask how often they visited their chiropractor. The answer is usually the same, "four or five times."

When a person goes to the gym to get into shape, results are not obtained nor maintained in just four or five visits. Time and commitment are required to achieve and maintain physical fitness. Correcting subluxations and keeping the spine at optimal health also requires time and a team effort between a patient and his or her doctor of chiropractic.

Is It Too Late?

If a patient's spine has been misaligned for years causing nerve interference, it could still be possible to achieve a healthy state. It would require the patient receive consistent chiropractic care and do his or her part by living a healthy lifestyle.

When the spine cannot move properly due to subluxation, the nervous system can be greatly affected. The nervous system controls and coordinates all body functions. It also helps the body relate and adapt to its environment.

When the spine is subluxated, communication from the nervous system to the body's organs, muscles and tissue can be interrupted. This can stop a person from reaching optimal health. I believe the answer to wellness cannot be found alone in drugs, surgery, diet or attitude, but by also having a healthy spine.

When Does Healing Begin?

With chiropractic, the healing begins when the spine is adjusted and subluxations are removed. This allows the nervous system to communicate freely.

Initially, the spine may need adjustments several times a week to remove the subluxations. Then, to keep the spine and nervous system healthy, spinal maintenance is necessary.

What About Injury?

Once the spine is injured, the degenerative process could begin. This could result in arthritis of the spinal joints.

Consider people who have played contact sports such as football, boxing or rugby. Think of those who have been in car accidents. These individuals may live with subluxations. If they have no pain and have not visited a chiropractor, they could be completely unaware their spine is degenerating.

Would you agree your health is your most valuable asset? Does this grab your attention and have you wanting to assure you have a healthy spine?

An Apple a Day?

Let us consider a person with tooth decay. He or she could believe his or her mouth is healthy unless pain is present.

Does a person only brush his or her teeth once and only brush again when pain arises? The answer is obviously no. If this were the case, by the time pain is felt, the decay process has already begun. We don't neglect our teeth. Neglecting the care of your spine could carry serious health consequences.

Unfortunately, most people are unaware the spine should be maintained throughout life to achieve optimal health.

Food, water, oxygen and nerve supply are necessary for sustaining life. I believe nerve supply is the body's number one priority. The spine provides protection. For this reason, would you agree it is important to ensure the spine is optimally maintained?

I urge you to visit a wellness chiropractor to have your spine checked for subluxations and begin the journey of wellnesscare! My family and I live a life of wellness. Twenty-first century chiropractic care is high-tech and high-touch producing high quality results for the whole family.

Chiropractic care could add *years to your life* and *life to your years*!

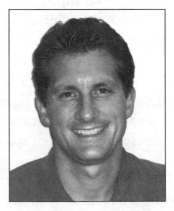

Dr. Robert C. Dees, D.C., RT
Canyon Chiropractic
San Ramon, CA
925-867-1414
A family wellness center specializing in
corrective chiropractic care

PART EIGHT

REGULAR CHIROPRACTIC CHECKUPS = A HEALTHY SPINE

By Dr. Matthew Lewis, D.C.

Have you ever noticed children today seem to have fewer cavities than their parents and grandparents?

How many people do you know with dentures these days?

Dentistry has made great strides in patient education during the last century, which has promoted good dental health and overall patient well-being.

It was different in the early 1900s. Then, when someone actually *went* to a dentist, it was at the point when his or her teeth were in terrible shape. Most of the time, a patient's teeth needed to be extracted. Dental care was not widely practiced at home. Even fewer people understood the impact of good dental health on the rest of the body.

Most of us would never dream of not taking our children, or ourselves, to the dentist! We teach our children to brush their teeth and how to floss. Dentists find fewer cavities in the mouths of kids today because good dental hygiene is practiced at home.

I believe chiropractic care is, today, where dentistry was 100 years ago. We learned how the care of our teeth affects our overall health. Chiropractic patients are finding spines free of subluxations contribute to wellness throughout their lives.

Subluxation is misalignment of the spine that causes pressure on the nerves. This pressure can result in many conditions adversely affecting overall health.

Like dentists during the early 20th century, I usually don't see patients until their health problems and pains have become severe. Most are very sick. Often they've seen every doctor in town, visited lots of different specialists and chiropractic is their last hope.

If they only knew after their car accident 20 years ago that chiropractic care could have helped to prevent problems they are having today!

Impact or trauma can cause subluxation that places pressure on the spinal cord and affects the nerves. Subluxation can cause a huge variety of health problems, including pain in various parts of the body.

Spills, Bumps and Bruises

A common misconception among people is the trauma they suffered has to be severe to hurt them.

I see patients in my office with subluxations. After I inquire, they remember falls, tumbles or minor vehicle accidents. At the time, they didn't think they were hurt because they didn't feel any pain.

The reality was the impact *did* affect their spines – they just didn't know it. With age, the symptoms of the subluxation could become more and more pronounced.

Most patients I see experienced not only a recent accident, but have weathered multiple traumas throughout their lives. That's probably true of most of us – football injuries 30 years ago, a fall off the porch when we were children or minor traffic accidents in our 20's.

All of these events could have unknowingly created adverse effects on our spines. Without treatment and as we grow older, they could affect our health. Patients rarely relate their condition to the accidents they may have had long ago.

With new patients, we start examinations with spinal x-rays

and lots of questions including what traumas may have caused damage. We can tell a lot just by looking at a patient's posture – in my opinion, posture is the window to the spine. With a program of specific adjustments, traction and exercise, many of my patients have had their subluxations corrected and their health restored.

Some patients try chiropractic years after the traumas occurred and are still capable of reaching near full correction. Some can live symptom-free and enjoy a better quality of life.

One of the most common subluxation patterns we see is the loss of normal curvature in the neck. This subluxation could be very serious because it may have a snowball effect on the entire body. Not only is the spine itself weakened, the spinal cord is stretched. This stretching affects all the nerves in the spinal column, which radiate to all areas of the body.

Even with a serious subluxation pattern such as this, chiropractic care results could be dramatic. But it doesn't happen overnight. Many times people come to my office for their first visits very discouraged. Many are barely able to work. It's difficult for them to lead productive lives.

Amazing transformations could take place after subluxations are corrected. Quality of life may improve significantly.

I've seen cases where lives have turned around because better health made patients happier people. Hopeless patients, who live with pain or health problems, might find they improve so much they start taking pleasure in life again. They might, once again, enjoy old activities they had given up or take on new challenges thought impossible.

I've seen patients improve from not just headaches, neck pain and back pain but also hearing problems, poor vision, dizziness, low energy, sleeping difficulty, balance problems, numbness, allergies and asthma. More importantly, they improved in mind, body and spirit and enjoy life again.

Although the results of correcting subluxation can be remarkable, I look forward to a day when prevention, just like dental care today, keeps people from enduring the pain and suffering of having unhealthy spines.

I've seen some tough cases of people in their teens and 20's. But the majority of my patients are in their 40's, 50's and 60's.

Trauma

People need to be aware any trauma, whether they feel pain associated with it or not, could affect the spine. Chiropractic care after the trauma could correct subluxation before additional problems occur. Even with the absence of pain at the time of injury, the spine could be degenerating on the inside.

We need to become more aware of what happens to us during a trauma.

You could fall, hurt your leg and be totally unaware your head bounced when you hit the ground. People need to be informed. I believe it is important to be checked by a chiropractor after any vehicle accident or fall.

I also encourage patients to bring in their children. Lots of injury-causing subluxations start in childhood. Children who are adjusted may not see the effects that could show up later.

I have entire families who come in for their adjustments together.

It usually starts with one of the adults having a problem and achieving successful results. After he or she experiences improved health and quality of life, he or she understands the importance of having a healthy spine.

He or she encourages the spouse to come, as well as bringing the children. This preventative care, just like the twice-a-year trips to the dentist, will have a big impact on the lives of the children as they grow older.

Like dentists 100 years ago, it's important for us to educate this generation, the next generation and the one after about taking care of their spines.

I can't wait to see the day when it's commonplace for entire families to visit chiropractors. I believe there will be less sickness and suffering. I feel my mission would be accomplished.

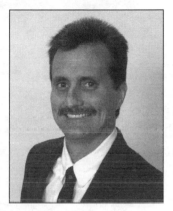

Dr. Matthew Lewis, D.C.
Lewis Chiropractic Center
Ocala, FL
352-861-0566

FOUNDATIONS FOR HEALTH

∾

By Dr. Daniel K. Claps, D.C.

Health could be defined as the condition when all the functions of the body, mind and spirit are normal and active. The basis of health is wellness, which is comprised of six components. Chiropractic supports wellness by improving the body's energy flow. Ideally, chiropractic is practiced proactively, often preventing ill health, rather than a reactive way of dealing with illness or the absence of health.

The Six Components of Wellness

There are six components or elements that work together to create wellness for an individual:

1. Proper exercise. Ninety minutes, three times a week can contribute to keeping the body in shape and toned. This exercise would consist of 30 minutes of cardio-vascular work, 30 minutes of stretching and 30 minutes of isotonic exercise with free weights or on machines.
2. Good posture. This reduces the stress on the spinal nerves and muscles.
3. Nutrition. We are what we absorb into our bodies. Today, in addition to good food, good nutrition requires good supplementation.
4. Good sleep. Generally six to eight hours every night allows the body to heal while we rest.

5. Positive mental attitude. It is very difficult to achieve health and wellness unless a person desires and believes they are possible.
6. Balanced spine. I believe this is the foundation of wellness because it controls the body's functions.

A chiropractor, acting as your health coach, can help you bring all six elements together in a way to support your total being.

Wellness Can Begin at Conception

Ideally, the chiropractic approach starts with parents who are drug-free and alcohol-free conceiving a child in an atmosphere of love and mutual support. Children conceived and born in this way have a huge head start on wellness. Their immune systems are not compromised by drugs or stress.

My wife, Maria, and I are committed to natural childbirth. Our first son was born in a birthing center with the help of a midwife.

We decided we wanted to have our second child at home. We began working with a wonderful midwife who was willing to support us in our home birth. At the time, she lived in Long Island, NY and we lived on Staten Island – about 45 minutes apart during non-commute hours.

On November 24, 1993, Maria awoke at about 3:15 a.m. with contractions coming every 10 minutes. I called our midwife. She asked me to call her back when Maria's contractions were five minutes apart. By 7:30 that morning, Maria's contractions were occurring every five minutes. When I reported this to our midwife, she agreed to come right over.

At about the same time, Maria's mother arrived to pick up our youngest. Looking at her daughter, she suggested we call 911. After reassuring my mother-in-law and walking her to her car, I rushed upstairs to find Maria on all fours, declaring she felt a huge urge to push. Glancing at my watch, I saw it was about 8:15. I wondered why our midwife hadn't arrived yet.

"It's too early," I thought as I tried to make Maria more comfortable. More in tune with the stage of her labor than I, Maria ordered me to go wash my hands.

I did.

When I returned, she was in active labor.

At her suggestion, I hurried to get the shower curtains we had purchased in preparation for the home birth. As gently as I could, I moved them beneath her hips to protect the bedding and provide a clean surface for the birth. As I did so, I realized the bag of water, which I knew was actually around the baby's head, was beginning to crown.

A quick call to our midwife, who was stuck in the height of the morning commute, confirmed my worst fears. She said, "You'll be doing this one. Good luck. I'll be there as soon as I can."

She went on to instruct me to break the bag of water.

Turning to my wife, I realized I didn't have any instruments. First, I gently poked at the crowning bag, and nothing happened. I knew I had to do something quickly. I found an area near my son's neck where the bag was loose. I gently pinched and tore at it. Within moments, I heard his cry as he moved from the birth canal into my waiting arms.

Placing my son on my wife's belly, I watch her go from pain to pure joy and back to pain again. The cord was still attached and pulling on her uterus. I clamped off the cord in two places and snipped it. Maria's pain eased immediately.

Our midwife arrived and complemented me profusely on helping with the birth. I was moved to write this poem:

Two hearts beating together
We are separated in an instant.
The awkwardness of the moment pierced only by the cry of life
Still yet attached...
Warmth is received at her side
I hold this precious one

Thanking God for what He has created in us and making it possible for us to experience it alone, quietly at home.

Several weeks later, a copy of Joel's birth certificate arrived. I was delighted to see my name as the birth attendant. I was dismayed to see the form had boxes for medical doctors, nurses, midwives, but none for doctors of chiropractic.

The point of this story is to demonstrate the natural process of childbirth. A woman's body is designed to carry and birth a baby. I believe children born in this natural way, with no drugs in their system because their mother has received no anesthesia, surrounded by family and love, begin their lives with wonderful foundations for wellness.

The Growth of Health Immune Systems

I believe chiropractic care is a strong approach to encourage the body's natural immune system, whether for an infant or an adult. I feel chiropractic care is so effective because the removal of subluxation through adjustments could restore the natural flow of life force. Such care could stimulate the immune system and organs such as the thymus gland, the lymph nodes, the spleen, the Peyer's Patches and the appendix.

The Essentials of Life

Chiropractic care not only can lead to true wellness, it can put us in touch with the essentials of life. Let me close with another poem that expresses how I see those essentials:

This is my daily bread
This is my daily water
This is my daily breath
This is my daily nerve supply
I am alive; I live for You daily.

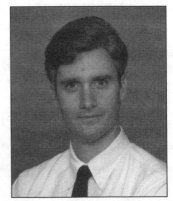

Dr. Daniel K. Claps, D.C.
Chiropractic Wellness Center
Brooklyn, NY
718-232-2225

PART TEN

LIVING HEALTHY WITH MORE ENERGY AND LESS STRESS

❧

By Dr. Thomas Potigian, D.C.

Growing up, I was extremely fortunate when it came to my health. While most kids saw a medical doctor for sickness and injuries, I was taken to see the family chiropractor. I was raised to understand and believe we have dynamic, bioelectrical and self-healing bodies. Having experienced the benefits of chiropractic firsthand, I knew very young I wanted to be a chiropractor.

I graduated from chiropractic college in December of 1981 and started practicing in 1982. I am committed to help patients achieve wellness by educating them about the miraculous benefits of a healthy spine and nervous system.

The body is created with internal energy (innate intelligence). Since the body's cells are constantly breaking down and regenerating, internal energy is necessary for body function.

The body's level of bioelectricity could fluctuate when a person becomes sick or injured. When energy of the body is its highest, optimal health is achieved.

If a person is aware his or her levels are decreasing, he or she has the opportunity to appropriately take action to increase them. Reducing mental and physical stress, getting proper rest and seeing a chiropractor could be included as examples of how to increase energy flow.

Subluxations cause pressure on the nerve system, which could interfere with the brain's communication to the rest of the body. In my opinion, to have an optimal functioning body with optimal health this energy flow must be at a maximum. The biggest problem affecting a body's energy flow is subluxation, which could cause a lowered state of health.

Three main types of stress affect the body. The first is emotional and mental stress, which can be triggered from working a demanding job or a death in the family. The next is physical stress, such as trauma to the body from a car accident or other types of injuries. Finally, chemical stress can occur when a person has a poor diet or takes medication.

Being around a negative environment or negative people could be very stressful on the body's physiology. Have you ever noticed you feel drained when around negative thinking people? Perhaps you have heard someone constantly saying negative things such as "you're ugly," "you're too skinny" or "you're too fat." These negative conversations could be very draining and even harmful to the body's physiology.

If the immune system is already weakened, a further decline could cause the body to be less capable of fighting infection.

The Power of Action

Exercise, in addition to chiropractic care, could help the body reduce the results of stress. When the body is under physical and mental stress, adrenalin production is increased. Without exercise, the adrenalin could remain at a high level for many days.

Adrenalin can cause a chemical acceleration in the body including heart rate.

Exercise causes an increase in circulation, metabolism and muscle contraction. This could help reduce or eliminate high levels of unnecessary adrenalin and increase levels of endorphins.

Endorphins create relaxation and comfort along with a decrease in pain. This results in a sense of euphoria during and after exercise.

Just as exercise is important for a person's optimal health, so is the intake of food. Eating too large a quantity of food in one sitting could cause the body's energy reserve to be utilized for digestion instead of mental function, possibly causing a state of lethargy. I believe it is best to eat smaller quantities of easily digestible foods more often versus one or two large meals.

The Adaptable You

The body is designed with the ability to adapt to the current environment. For example, when the body is cold, it shivers to generate heat. When the body is too hot, it sweats to cool itself down.

When a person is sick, the body's temperature could rise. This is how a fever begins. This normal response causes an increase in circulation, respiration and metabolism so the body may effectively fight infection.

These are all normal functions of a body adapting and healing. If a person takes an aspirin to lower a fever, the body's ability to overcome the illness could be reduced.

Most doctors understand damage to the spinal cord could cause or lead to paralysis such as quadriplegia. Equally important and more common could be pressure on the nerve root or mechanoreceptors in the spine. Pressure to the nerve root could cause abnormal function of the tissue and organs of the body due to communication interference within the nervous system.

The New You

The body is constantly regenerating. This means old cells are replaced by new cells. The process of regeneration involves every organ and cell within the body. The nerve system is an important part of the regeneration and healing processes.

When physical, emotional or chemical stress occurs, subluxation within the nervous system could develop causing interference in the regeneration process, possibly leading to disease.

The brain controls the body. The spinal cord and nerves are the pathways for information to travel from the brain. Eliminating stress by removing subluxations could be paramount to optimal health.

Unfortunately, many people are not aware of how subluxations occur. They give little thought to how stress and trauma could affect their bodies.

A great example is a patient of mine who was in such extreme pain he could only sleep two hours each night while in a recliner. As part of consultations and examinations, I ask my patients about past traumas. In this particular case, I asked this man if he had any past injuries or trauma.

He replied, "No."

After 20 minutes, he recalled having a bus hit him, a brick thrown from a four-story building strike him on the head and a bomb blow up in front of him.

After examining him and taking an x-ray, I found this patient was in desperate need of chiropractic care. His traumas were more than 30 years old. Stress and subluxations had been affecting his body for that entire time. The effects and damage to his spine and the nerve pressure would require time to correct. I explained it would take a minimum of one year to correct and rehabilitate his spine and nerve system. After a year of adjusting his spine, he was once again able to get a full night's sleep in bed with minimal discomfort.

The problem often is, without pain, people consider themselves healthy. I believe health is based on how the body functions on the inside. The liver, kidneys and gallbladder cannot be felt. Yet, they could be in a diseased state. Absence of symptoms does not mean a body is healthy.

God created this amazing body with capability of healing itself. I feel, with proper health discipline and maintenance, the body can live without disease. Be aware of the three major forms of stress. Include regular chiropractic care in your life. By taking better care of yourself, you could live a longer, healthier life…possibly seeing 100 years old.

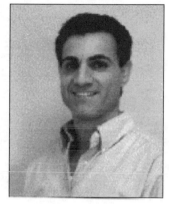

Dr. Thomas Potigian, D.C.
Sunnyside Chiropractic Center
Fresno, CA
559-454-1000
teampotigian@aol.com
www.sunnysidechiropractic.com
Dr. Potigian specializes in spinal
corrective care.

CHAPTER FIVE

THE DRAMATIC DIFFERENCE WHEN SUBLUXATIONS ARE REMOVED

PART ONE

BACK ON TOP

❦

By Dr. Amy E. Orta, D.C. and Dr. Jose L. Orta, D.C.

At 24 years old, I worked for a New York based company making a great amount of money for a new college grad. I was considered a "star-performer" climbing the financial ladder of success.

I worked long, hard hours and played just as hard. My husband and I skied in the mountains of Vermont during the winter weekends. We played on the private beaches of Breezy Point in the summer. We sailed, swam scuba and played beach volleyball. You name it; we did it! We were young and newly married riding a fabulous wave of success.

Who knew how quickly it could end? We were only married one year and one day when I was in a car accident.

After the immediate injuries were handled, I searched for months trying to find someone to help me deal with the physical and emotional outcome of the accident. There wasn't a medical professional or therapist I could find in New York who could help me. My life withered away one piece at a time.

I thought, for sure, God had forsaken me.

The pain was so excruciating, I could hardly lift a dinner plate. It felt as if a thousand knives were stabbing my joints, muscles and withering body.

My husband and I divorced. Everything I knew to be good, right and true appeared in my mind as an old movie repeating itself without a happy ending.

I ultimately lost my desire to live. I actually considered the different ways I could end my life. I thought the simplest would be to overdose. I had no drive and no hope. I hurt physically and emotionally. I decided that week would be my last.

Then, a miracle happened.

In Duluth, Georgia there was a chiropractor whom I believe God brought to me. The doctor managed to remove interferences within my body. He told me this type of care was called "Specific Chiropractic Adjustment." I was told this care would remove something in my spine called vertebral subluxation.

I felt better after the removal of these vertebral subluxations. It was truly amazing!

By removing these subluxations, or misalignments of the bones in my back, my body was able to reconnect to my brain. My life line was turned back on. My life restored.

My mind became clear. My body became strong. My spirit began to express its God given full life potential once again!

I thank God for helping me discover and receive chiropractic care.

Even today, I receive chiropractic adjustments. This allows me to maintain a strong physical and spiritual life. Trauma along with physical, mental and emotional daily stresses caused my subluxations. I will not allow life's daily hassles to subluxate me ever again.

I decided to reenter college and become a chiropractor. I wanted to save the lives of others faced with challenges.

I've been blessed with a new life. My husband, Dr. Jose, is also a doctor of chiropractic. As he has expressed to me time and time again, "God can make all things new." He is absolutely right.

When Dr. Jose was 18-years-old, he was on his high school

swim team. He dove head first into the pool and hit bottom. Incredibly, he swam up dazed and in pain. He was too proud and embarrassed to tell anyone what happened.

Three years passed before Jose saw his first symptoms.

His condition manifested as tingling down his arm. Then, he lost sensation. Next, he lost strength. Pain increased. His back and chest tightened with a vise-like grip.

He decided to "work it out" in the gym. He thought daily workouts would help him regain strength.

Shortly after, Jose woke and rolled over in bed. His arm did not follow. Motionless, lifeless, paralysis had set. As most people would have done, he sought the care of a medical doctor.

The medical doctor had mistakenly diagnosed Jose with Carpel Tunnel Syndrome. He offered Jose two choices.

One choice was consuming increasing amounts of prescription pain killers and muscle relaxants.

Option two was surgery.

By the grace of God, Jose ran into a family friend who had attended college to become a doctor of chiropractic. They began to talk. The friend told Jose there was a third option which did not require drugs or surgery. It made sense; Jose believed God didn't create us deficient of pain killers and muscle relaxants.

Without really knowing what the chiropractor could do to help, but with no other desirable options, Jose gave chiropractic a try.

Miraculously, within less than 4 weeks, his arm started to come back to life. The tingling had subsided. Sensation began to return. His strength intensified.

Together with a Mission

Together, with God as our guide, Jose and I have a mission: To assist in bringing people back in connection with God.

You see, we believe only God could have given new life to two such destroyed bodies and made them thrive.

Mind, Body and Spirit Family Chiropractic is the name of our practice. We believe wellness is the ability of mind, body and spirit to express God's will 100% of the time without interference.

We educate our patients about the holistic and all natural principles and philosophies of chiropractic. We share the science we acquired while earning our doctorates including anatomy, physiology and neurology. We illustrate the technical art of adjusting the spine to remove vertebral subluxations, which can stop communication between the brain and body.

Personally, we maintain our health by maintaining our spines. We believe God expresses Himself through human thoughts, actions and words. For optimal communication, we must maintain our bodies clear of nerve interference.

The most common nerve interference comes from misalignment of spinal bones. Chiropractic checkups make sure the spine is aligned and is the best way to be certain the body is working 100% of the time without nerve interference.

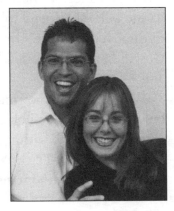

Dr. Jose L. Orta, D.C.
Dr. Amy E. Orta, D.C.
Mind, Body & Spirit Chiropractic, Inc.
Fort Lauderdale, FL
954-489-4790
chiropracticmbs@aol.com
www.mbschiropractic.com
Dr. Jose and Dr. Amy practice
family wellnesscare.

PART TWO

IS YOUR BODY GETTING WHAT IT NEEDS?

◈

By Dr. Anthony Bastecki, D.C.

The benefits of chiropractic have been a part of my life since I was a young child.

Arriving home from school with my brothers and sister, it was dark and silent – no lights, no television and no stereo.

It wasn't because my dad forgot to pay the electric bill. It meant my father was suffering from another debilitating migraine headache. His headaches were so painful; he would lie in the dark in total silence for days.

Can you imagine four kids being silent for days?

My father's medication became increasingly stronger. At times, he existed as a deranged zombie. Regardless of the medication strength, he had little relief. Medication was certainly no cure. The doctor finally told my father, "It's all in your head."

After a long, futile search for relief, a friend convinced my father to give chiropractic a try.

The chiropractor performed an exam, took some x-rays and then "adjusted" my dad's spine. The adjustment didn't hurt. In fact, my dad said it actually felt good. But most importantly, my dad felt relief from the migraines which had plagued him his whole life. He became a new person – fun and loving. It changed my family life.

With my dad's great results, our entire family became chiropractic patients. We still are today. My brother and I witnessed such a positive impact for our family, we each attended chiropractic school.

My dad's painful condition illustrates what can happen when nerve supply, one of the four essentials of life, is compromised.

The scientific community acknowledges there are four basic essentials to life including food, water, air and nerve supply. Without anyone one of these, you could not exist. If just one were negatively altered, you would experience a detrimental affect on your life and health.

Optimizing these essentials daily can have a direct influence on your optimal health.

Is Your Body Really Getting What it Needs?

An overwhelming amount of information exists on the four essentials.

Food, for example, has been extensively researched. New information continues to surface almost daily. It is common knowledge certain diets have beneficial results on different health problems and conditions.

The importance of water to our health also has been thoroughly examined. There is an abundance of information on the quantities and quality of fluids we should consume daily.

As for oxygen, the positive effect of aerobic activity in increasing vital lung capacity and oxygenation of tissue is also well known.

This brings us to nerve supply. While this may be the area with some of the most in-depth research and information, it is also the least understood by the general public and the non-research community. Nerve supply is the key area where chiropractic can play an important role in optimizing your health.

Let's look at what chiropractic is, what it does, its benefits and the part it plays in the body's total health picture.

Chiropractic focuses on the spinal column and its effect on the vital components of the nervous system.

Minor misalignments of the spine can occur. These are known as vertebral subluxations. Subluxations can irritate the nervous system and affect the functional capabilities of the body.

Some people refer to this as having a "pinched nerve." The problem is that the word "pinched" is generally associated with pain. The fact is that few nerves – less than 10 percent – carry pain signals. This means serious spinal damage could be present and go undetected because there is no accompanying pain.

Subluxation, Itself, Has No Symptoms

Symptoms may arise later resulting from the tissue damage developed over time. Regular spinal evaluations for early detections of subluxation are highly recommended. Like most health problems, the earlier you find this condition, the easier it is to correct.

What should you do if subluxation is detected in your spine? Your chiropractor will likely perform a scientifically designed sequence of corrective spinal adjustments. Then, he or she may recommend exercises, stretches and specific corrective traction to help stabilize the associated spinal soft tissue.

A properly aligned spine is structurally and functionally stable resulting in an optimally functioning nervous system.

A July 15, 2003, clinically controlled study published in *Spine,* authored by Dr. Reinhold Muller, PhD and Dr. Lynton G.F. Giles, DC, PhD, showed the superiority of chiropractic care for chronic lower back pain over acupuncture and medication.

The study was conducted at a hospital's multidisciplinary spinal pain unit between February 1999 and October 2001 with 115 patients. One group of patients was given chiropractic care. Another group was treated with acupuncture. A third group received the drugs Celebrex (200-400mg/day) and Vioxx (12.5-25mg/day).

The study concluded "for chronic spinal pain syndromes, it

appears that spinal manipulation (chiropractic adjustments) proved the best overall short-term results..."

The study also stated, "Even though the chiropractic care group was the most chronic (the average duration of spinal pain symptoms was 8.3 years compared to 6.4 years for the medication group and 4.5 years for the acupuncture group), 27.3% recovered with 18 spinal adjustments over a period of 9 weeks, or less." This is compared to 9.4% who recovered with acupuncture and 5% recovery with medications.

Now that I've shared what chiropractic can do, ask yourself, "Is my body really getting what it needs?"

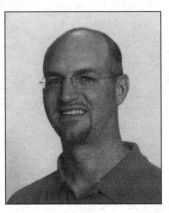

Dr. Anthony Bastecki, D.C.
Bastecki Chiropractic
Lexington, KY
859-266-2223

PART THREE

BLESSINGS IN DISGUISE

~≋~

*By Dr. Barbara Hannam, D.C.
and Dr. Dwayne Hannam, D.C.*

We started in chiropractic in similar ways. As Barbara tells her story:

When I was 12 years old, I fell down a set of stairs. Even though nothing was broken, I found myself in debilitating pain long after the initial stiffness passed. Fortunately, my family took me to a chiropractor. The care worked.

While under care, I began to realize people were there for many reasons. They were all getting help. Later in my teens, I worked part time in a chiropractor's office. Again, I saw how chiropractic care helped create many positive life changes. I entered chiropractic school because I have always wanted to help people. Dwayne and I met on the first day of chiropractic classes.

Dwayne shares his story:

I too came to chiropractic through an injury. It happened while playing basketball in high school. I was clipped. I landed hard, face-first on the floor shattering teeth and splitting my chin wide open. I was rushed to the emergency room. After hours of waiting, the doctor stitched me, gave me drugs for pain and suggested I see a dentist.

For the next four and a half years, I suffered from pneumonia at least two to three times per year, without realizing this may be due to the fall. I could no longer participate in sports. It was all I could do to keep up with my studies.

Traditional doctors could only offer drugs. I was close to despair when a friend suggested chiropractic care. I blew him off.

In my second year at the university, I was at a job fair. There was a chiropractor with a plastic spine. He was using it for demonstration purposes. I asked him what he could do for me.

He replied, "If the brain sends its signals to the body through the spinal cord and attaching nerves, doesn't it make sense if the spine, which protects these communication lines, is out of alignment it might distort the signals? Maybe that distortion is the actual source of why you're having so many problems with your lungs."

That made sense to me. The doctor went on to explain how corrective care could remedy the misalignments and restore the natural energy flow. I began a course of care that restored my health.

I'd known for years I wanted to help people. When I learned how this process took care of my breathing issues, I became a chiropractor. I met Barbara in the process.

Two Doctors; One Healing Message

In our family practice we start our wellness focus by emphasizing the importance of posture. Your mother was right when she told you to stand up straight. She may have even tried to help your posture by telling you to practice walking with a book balanced on your head. Although she probably didn't understand the science behind it, she was going in the right direction.

Posture actually reflects your overall body function. This bold statement is supported by research published in the *American Journal of Pain Management*, Volume 4, No. 1, January 1994. The study concludes on page 39, "Posture affects all human function, both consciously and unconsciously, from breathing to thinking."

When your spine is aligned properly, your nervous system and its vital energy flow can function better. Your immune system could be strengthened. Your vital organs could function at more optimal levels.

What happens when your spine is out of alignment? The energy flow from your brain, through your spinal cord and nerves, to your major organs and the rest of your body could become distorted. This reduces your body's ability to optimally heal and perform.

You can observe this yourself. Take a look at the people around you. Notice if people's shirts are level on their shoulders. If you see their shoulders aren't level, you know they could have a problem. Look and see if their heads are forward or off balance.

Now, notice the difference in the energy. People who are walking tall and balanced seem to have more energy than those who don't.

Poor posture could also have a negative impact on breathing. According to Rene Cailliet, MD, and Leonard Gross in their book, *The Rejuvenation Strategy* (Doubleday, 1987), "Poor posture depletes your pulmonary capacity by as much as 30%."

With a chiropractor helping you, could you and your family move toward better health?

As part of our evaluation process, we often use a bilateral scale to measure weight symmetry from the left side of the body to the right side. Ideally, the difference between the two sides should be no more than about five pounds. However, we often observe a variation of as much as 30 to 40 pounds. We combine this information with x-rays, which act as valuable blueprints to objectively evaluate and follow patients' care. This allows patients to experience a better quality of health care by having the ability to view individual progress.

We are delighted when our patients tell us how much better they feel as their postures improve. It's not surprising to us that energy flow increases from the brain to the body as posture improves.

However, we are quick to point out gauging your health only by how you feel could be misleading.

You may not feel a heart attack coming on ten years prior to the attack. By not feeling it you might falsely believe you are healthy while this devastating process could be progressing in your body.

The Path to Wellness

Chiropractic care involves the correction of subluxation. Subluxation occurs when one of your spinal bones move out of its normal position placing pressure on or irritating a nerve. This pressure or irritation could disrupt the normal flow of energy from your brain to the rest of your body. Specific adjustments move the spine back towards normal with the goal of restoring or improving energy flow.

We work with whole families, including newborns and young children.

We are often asked why youngsters might need chiropractic care. We find ourselves suggesting parents observe their own children. Are they carrying large backpacks, usually on one shoulder? When children drop their backpacks, are their shoulders level and their postures good? If not, these are indications of the need for chiropractic care.

One of our favorite stories of success with children is the two-year-old who came to us diagnosed with autism. He was withdrawn and hypersensitive. Allopathic (traditional) medicine didn't offer his parents much hope.

We began a series of adjustments. Over time, he began to improve. We are delighted to report, at five-years-old, he was able to attend regular school and showed few signs of the original diagnosis.

The Three T's

Our goal is both corrective care and education. We talk with families about the three T's. Any one could cause subluxation and distort the energy flow through the body.

- Thought – The things we think about could have a huge effect on our health. Negative thoughts may actually cause physical damage. This includes thoughts of anxiety, stress and depression.
- Trauma – Injury is the most obvious way our spines might become misaligned.
- Toxins – Pollutants could include all sorts of things. These range from the obvious, like smog and cigarette smoke, to the chemicals in processed foods and even some medicines.

As our patients learn about their own bodies and experience regular chiropractic care, they are able to move toward optimum health.

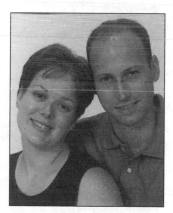

Dr. Barbara Hannam, D.C.
Dr. Dwayne Hannam, D.C.
Cranberry Chiropractic
Middleboro, MA
508-947-6455

PART FOUR

THE HEALER WITHIN

❧

By Dr. Mark Lagerkvist, D.C.

We were born with amazing capability. Our bodies were created with the ability to heal themselves. From the moment of our conception until we take our final breath, our bodies are constantly engaged in the process of renewal. This innate function of regenerating life force is what I call "the healer within."

It all begins with the brain…

The brain directs and controls every function of the body. It sends its instructions, information and impulses through the spinal cord and nerves to every cell.

Like a garden hose watering a garden, the spinal cord irrigates the body, via the nerves, with life-sustaining information from the brain. The uninhibited flow of this information keeps the body functioning in optimal health.

But through the course of everyday life, the nerves can become blocked. This could interrupt the brain-body connection and choke the electrical energy needed to sustain the body's balance of health and well-being.

Imagine stepping on a garden hose. What happens to the flow of water?

Now, think of your spinal cord and nerves. What would happen if the same type of pressure was applied? The resulting pressure on the nerves and spinal cord interrupts or stops the flow of information from your brain. Just like the garden needs water, your body's cells need information from your brain to function correctly.

When subluxation causes interference between the brain and body, optimal health is compromised. The body experiences *disease*. And, as it progresses, symptoms begin to appear.

Now, this is a concept which seems to contradict conventional wisdom. This is a central principle of chiropractic care: Symptoms occur *after* the disease process has begun.

Often, by the time you feel any physical symptoms, the disease has already progressed.

Dentists have known this for years. By the time you feel the pain of the toothache, the decay has already taken over the root of the tooth.

Wellnesscare Focus

Chiropractors focus on maintaining wellness. With regular maintenance of the spine, many diseases of the body could be avoided. Doctors of chiropractic employ varying techniques to correct and prevent misalignments of the spine, facilitating the flow of regenerating impulses from the brain.

A chiropractor is specifically trained to locate and respond to advance warning signals. By freeing the natural flow of energy and communication between the brain and the organs, our bodies can do what they were designed to do – maintain themselves in optimal health.

It seems so simple, doesn't it? Yet, many people today have no idea what chiropractic care is all about. Simply put, chiropractic could help sick people get well and prevent the healthy from getting sick.

Imagine the amount of time and money people could save if we learned to let our bodies function as they were intended.

Society seems to be growing more disillusioned with treatment limitations, high healthcare costs and the growing risks associated with some forms of medical treatments. More and more people are seeking alternatives.

As people learn more about their bodies and realize "one-size-fits-all" medicine does not fit their needs, they are seeking more individual, natural care.

The ancient physician Hippocrates advised his students to learn as much as they possibly could about the workings of the spine. It is my understanding he said, within the spine they would find the origin of many diseases.

Chiropractic Thriving

Chiropractic has evolved into a thriving profession that is licensed, administered and accepted as a valid form of preventive or "wellness" healthcare worldwide.

As knowledge and understanding of the profession grows, and as patients discover the healing power that resides in their own bodies, the number of skeptics who dismiss chiropractic as "quackery" decreases. Only those who are uninformed slander its practice.

I speak from personal experience. A little more than fifteen years ago, I was a competitive swimmer for the University of Wisconsin. I traveled to competitions throughout the country as one of the top in my field. While training midway through my first year, I began to lose sensation from my shoulder to fingertips in my left arm ultimately losing pulse to that arm. I was unable to hold a toothbrush, turn a screwdriver or perform the simplest tasks.

The medical doctors diagnosed shoulder problems. They placed me on a series of fifteen different anti-inflammatory drugs. As each one wore off, I received a new prescription. I experienced drug side-effects, which in my opinion harmed my liver, kidneys, digestive and immune system. I became chronically ill.

Because anti-inflammatory drugs only mask the problem, I continued to train causing further damage to my body.

I wasn't getting any better. In fact, I was growing worse. The university hospital began running tests on me. They poked, prodded and scanned me. I felt like a guinea pig.

After many thousands of dollars worth of testing, I was told I needed to have a rib removed to make room for nerves, arteries and veins. I spent the next year and a half searching for a second, less drastic opinion. I saw the best specialists in the country only to be told the same thing at each office.

While searching for an alternative to surgery, I lost my swimming scholarship, neglected my studies, and alienated both family and friends. In an attempt to deal with the depression I was experiencing, I turned to alcohol.

I lost everything I had worked for during the previous twelve years. Finally, I decided to have the surgery, as there seemed no other recourse.

The surgery did not work. I continued my downward spiral into alcohol abuse and depression.

I was at rock bottom when my father recommended I try chiropractic. While skeptical, I listened to what the doctor had to say. It made so much sense.

Within the first couple of adjustments, the doctor was able to temporarily restore the blood and nerve flow to my left arm. From then on, I knew what I would do for the rest of my life. I would be a chiropractor committed to saving others lives just as I am convinced that doctor saved mine.

I don't know what caused the subluxation that resulted in my health problems. I do know if the alcohol hadn't killed me, the subluxation may have or lead to other health issues. To this day, I am checked weekly and adjusted, if necessary, in order to maintain the health God gave me.

I'm grateful for the knowledge I gained and the care that I received. And today I tell my own patients, "I move the bones; God does the healing. I'm not the healer; I simply support the process."

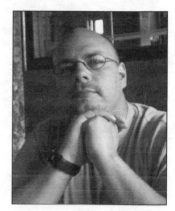

Dr. Mark Lagerkvist, D.C.
Lifeline Principled Chiropractic
Olympia Field, FL
708-481-5444
www.druglesshealing.net
www.askdoctormark.com

Dr. Mark Lagerkvist is a noted chiropractor, consultant, lecturer and seminar leader. He is committed to helping people transform their minds, bodies and souls through Life Works Ltd. Life Works offers Life Works Consulting, Life Line Chiropractic, Life Path Retreats and Seminars, Life Essentials Luxury Supplements and Life Works Financial. All of these support human beings in discovering and fulfilling their missions.

PART FIVE

CHIROPRACTIC AWARENESS: A JOURNEY TO OPTIMUM HEALTH

By Dr. Beth Ehlich, D.C. and Dr. Chris Ehlich, D.C.

We believe chiropractic is becoming America's most recognized form of complimentary health care with twenty-five million patients every year. Yet, some people still wonder exactly how chiropractic can heal and miss its potential benefits.

Contrary to a popular misconception, chiropractic goes beyond the assessment and treatment of musculoskeletal dysfunction.

Chiropractic care can be a journey toward greater health, wellness and spiritual awareness. It can provide true healing in all areas of our lives. For many chiropractors, including ourselves, chiropractic is a life purpose.

Dr. Beth suffered greatly from sinus and allergy problems as a teenager and chronic severe ear infections from infancy throughout childhood. We met just before her senior year in high school and began dating.

Dr. Chris saw how great Beth's suffering was and encouraged Beth to seek chiropractic care with his parents, Drs. Bruce and Judy Ehlich. After determining the cause was an atlas subluxation, Beth received her first adjustment at the age of 17.

Since then, with regular chiropractic care, Dr. Beth enjoys a higher level of health and is totally free from the ailments that were a part of her growing up. Chiropractic has allowed Dr. Beth to express her full potential for health.

Dr. Beth cannot imagine life without adjusts from her chiropractor who, as the Lord would have it, is Dr. Chris.

If not for chiropractic, Dr. Beth feels her life today would be plagued by other severe sufferings that would have drastically lowered the quality of her life. Chiropractic changed her life. The change was so evident that she wanted to share it with other people. This is why Dr. Beth is a chiropractor today: to help those suffering needlessly to restore their health.

Overcoming Challenges Through Wellness

We feel wellness is an optimal state in which the body is equipped physically, mentally, emotionally and spiritually to respond to major health and life challenges. During this state, a person is able to express their full health potential.

We believe chiropractic is the key ingredient to attaining and maintaining this state of wellness. It offers fascinating insights into the complex relationship between mind, emotions and body. It can also reveal how we could use these insights to achieve greater health and harmony.

The term "chiropractic" (from Greek for "done by hand") was conceived in 1895 by the profession's founder, Daniel David Palmer, in Davenport, Iowa. Chiropractic is concerned with the restoration and preservation of health. It focuses particular attention on subluxations which can occur anywhere in the spine.

Vertebral subluxations consist of functional, structural or pathological changes that can compromise neurological integrity. This may negatively influence organ system function and general health.

Chiropractors are trained to detect and correct vertebral subluxations with spinal adjustments and chiropractic procedures. For Americans who suffer from vertebral subluxations, chiropractic offers non-invasive, natural healing that could go beyond temporary relief to optimum healing and spinal function. A chiropractic adjustment administered to remove a subluxation can be gentle, low force and drug-free.

Chiropractic holistically combines specific spinal adjustments to remove nerve interference. Chiropractic works with the inherent intelligence within the body that guides our overall wellness. Chiropractors firmly believe the power that created the body can heal the body.

Education is the key to increasing public awareness about the enormous benefits of chiropractic care. Ignorance and lack of information can lead to prejudice, misconceptions and false fears. By educating the public about chiropractic, we hope to eliminate fears.

Chiropractic adjustments are pain-free and safe. They can be gentle with very little to no discomfort. Chiropractic side effects are extremely uncommon.

The use of some medications could interfere with the body's self-healing mechanisms and could lead to drug-caused diseases or complications. This awareness can motivate more people to take charge of their own health and become increasingly informed about available options. We recommend you always ask about long term affects of any care.

The increasing popularity of complementary and alternative health care has created a unique opportunity for chiropractic professionals to share their vision and expertise with local communities.

Many chiropractors, including ourselves, offer regular informational seminars to new patients and their families. In these seminars, we explain the basic principles of spinal health and the health increasing benefits of removing nervous system interferences caused by subluxation. The goal is to help patients achieve healthy, vibrant, energized lifestyles…the chiropractic way.

Knowledge of chiropractic benefits is growing. A growing number of orthopedic surgeons and general practitioners are encouraging patients to seek chiropractic care. As a result, an increasing number of people are choosing chiropractic for a drug-free approach to health and wellnesscare while relying on mainstream medicine for emergency treatment.

Without proper education, patients might discontinue chiropractic care when they feel better, they have fewer symptoms or results require time.

People who understand chiropractic tend to continue with our recommendations. They could become chiropractic patients for life. These individuals tend to pay more attention to the healing process and can feel changes gradually taking place within their bodies.

Subluxations at Birth

When women realize the possible traumas associated with the birth process, they understand how they and their children might have been affected.

Babies' first subluxations could occur during birth. The sooner a baby is checked for subluxations, the sooner any injury or stress from birth can be dealt with safely and gently. To achieve optimum health for ourselves and our children, we must make sure our bodies function the way they were meant with absolutely nothing interfering with the process.

Chiropractic could help you determine underlying causes for your children's illnesses. It provides a healing program that could produce lasting results.

Sometimes, we meet our patients a few days or even hours after they have been born. We find many people are committed to their children being checked early. They understand the importance of a healthy spine and want the best for their families.

A rewarding part of being a chiropractor is to witness the chiropractic results of children who no longer have to suffer, take medicine, spend time in hospitals or go through harmful procedures. When these children grow up, we would not be surprised to find their children receive chiropractic adjustments as well. We look forward to seeing several generations of people receiving adjustments regularly, which will lead to increasingly widespread chiropractic awareness in all parts of the world.

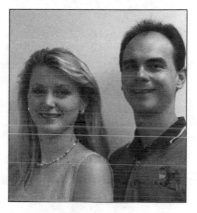

Dr. Beth Ehlich, D.C.
Dr. Chris Ehlich, D.C.
Ehlich Family Chiropractic
Greer, SC
864-848-3912

Dr. Beth and Dr. Chris are members of the All World Chiropractic Team. Dr. Chris serves as Vice President of the Palmetto State Chiropractic Association and the South Carolina State Representative of the International Chiropractors Association.

PART SIX

HOW I BECAME A DOCTOR OF CHIROPRACTOR – AN ANSWERED PRAYER

By Dr. Charles Nathaniel, D.C.

At 19 years old, I found myself confused and lacking direction.

My parents wanted me to go into the family business, but that held no appeal. I tried studying various things like film, English literature, even math and physics, but nothing clicked.

I decided travel would not only relieve the pressure I felt, but help me discover myself as well. Wanting the exotic, and the kinds of adventures I'd read about in so many of James Michener's novels, I headed east to India.

At first India was a cultural shock to me. I recoiled emotionally from the smells, sights and sounds that accosted me. With so many homeless people, the streets smelled like a public toilet that was never sanitized. Old men carted mountains of goods and young children collected dung for home cooking fires. Beggars, monkeys, and cows paraded through the streets.

Each night families would reclaim their spots on the streets and proceed to pick nits of lice from each other's scalps. Then they would sleep as best they could.

As I walked those streets staring at thousands of gazing eyes, I was filled with isolation and aloneness. Months later, despite the apparent squalor, I began to see the spirituality and resource-fulness. I sensed a whole different rhythm to life than I had ever imagined.

On my 20th birthday, I found myself in Goa on India's west coast. My feelings of separation intensified and tormented me. My emotions had been plaguing me for so long, without warning or control, I found myself crying out to God.

"God, these feeling of sadness and loneliness are killing me. Please guide me to do something worthy, something to help humanity. Something I can do with my hands because I don't want to be in an office pushing a pencil. Let me do something that will ease my soul and help me feel a greater connection to my fellow human beings. Please, God, please help me!"

Soon after praying, I became even more emotional and irrational. I could not tolerate food and could not sleep. For the better part of a week, I wandered the beaches of Goa. Early one dawn, I collapsed from exhaustion.

When I awoke I discovered my eyes and skin had turned yellow. I was ill with hepatitis and jaundice.

Hospitals in India were like nothing I had experienced in the west. I was in a large room that held about 30 simple cots. There were few doctors or nurses and not much medicine. Instead, each patient's family moved in to give the best care they could. They surrounded the sick person's cot all day and night, sleeping and eating wherever they found space. The constant activity, noise and heat drained me further.

Two cots away from me was a young man from California who also had hepatitis. He appeared much sicker than I. I could hardly believe what I saw. He was incoherently tossing and turning in attempts to rise from his cot. A young American couple attending him physically restrained him.

A day or so later, I awoke to discover his cot was empty. At first I thought he might have had a miraculous healing, but was soon informed he had died.

Witnessing the reality of death hit me hard. I was filled with a determination to live. I absolutely refused to die in India, leaving my parents in the painful position of receiving some bureaucratic notification of my death. My nights were filled with the sounds of coughing patients, yet in my dreams I saw myself living in a holy commune.

After two more weeks in the hospital, I couldn't take it any more. I was weak, had lost 29 pounds and wasn't getting any better. The dreams persisted. I demanded to be released and made my way to an ashram where I learned to meditate, prepare vegetarian food and trust my inner-self.

Some months later, I was able to return home to Montreal strong as ever. Glad to be home, I was eager to get on with my life, even though I still had no specific direction or career in mind.

I soon developed a physical condition my doctor thought, at first, was hives. Without warning, I would feel painful, needle-like pricking sensations and breakout in bumps.

Sometimes the pain and welts would be limited to one part of my body. Other times, the pricking sensation would rage all over. These attacks might happen once a day or 20 times a day.

All I could do when an episode started was try to remain calm and find a private place where I could wait for it to subside. Due to the frustrating nature of my condition, I abandoned any hopes of pursuing a normal social or academic life until my health would normalize.

The first doctor gave me medicine I was glad to take. It began to affect my stomach which ached and felt drum tight.

Before long, my doctor referred me to a specialist. I was actually on the specialist's examining table when an attack began. He watched what was happening to me and then commented, "Interesting."

He asked if he could bring in his colleagues to see what was going on. Soon there were four doctors checking me and scratching their heads.

Nine months later, I was told whatever was causing my problem was not life threatening. I should learn to live with my condition.

You may have heard the saying that when one door closes, another door opens. For me the opening was chiropractic.

At the time, I knew nothing about chiropractic but met and made an appointment with a doctor of chiropractic. The doctor examined, x-rayed and promised me a report the next day.

When I returned to his office, the doctor told me I had several subluxations or misalignments in my spine. The worst was at the seventh thoracic vertebra.

The doctor showed me a chart demonstrating how this vertebra affects the function of the liver. To my amazement, he described how the liver is a factory producing and storing vital chemicals the body requires to be released into the blood stream in exact amounts at precise times. The doctor also explained to me the skin is an organ of elimination.

The doctor believed the subluxation caused my liver to malfunction and caused my body to be toxic. The toxicity was eliminated through my skin. The hives were a terrible symptom of a toxic body.

This was a revelation to me, particularly since I had never mentioned my bout with hepatitis, which has been known to adversely affect the liver.

My doctor recommended a course of spinal adjustments at a frequency of three times a week for three months. With renewed hope, I decided to follow the care in full faith.

The first month, there was no change. I persisted because his explanations made sense.

During the second month, I thought I might be experiencing a slight lessening of my problem, but I wasn't sure.

By the end of the third month, I had totally recovered and have not suffered a trace since.

Going to a doctor of chiropractic was an educational experience. I met and spoke with many of the patients in the reception room. I discovered they were genuinely satisfied with their care and truly respected the doctor. They encouraged me by way of their results.

In addition, the doctor's staff taught me every spinal adjustment could facilitate healing of the body.

When I think back to my conversation with God, I realize He had a purpose for me. I became seriously ill to discover healing comes from within. I feel I was chosen to educate, serve and help people gain vitality.

For the past 26 years, I have been teaching my patients life is an expression of intelligence. Chiropractic promotes the body's natural ability to regulate and heal itself.

I also tell them to be mindful of what they pray. Prayers are meant to be answered, just as mine.

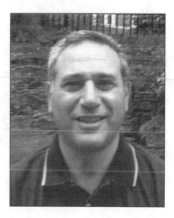

Dr. Charles Nathaniel, D.C.
West Island Chiropractic Center
Montreal, Quebec, Canada
514-694-6332
westchiro@yahoo.com

Dr. Charles Nathaniel, D.C., is proud to be a member of a profession that is made up of dedicated men and women whose work promotes healing and harmony for present and future generations.

"It is better to light one candle than to curse the darkness."
– B.J. Palmer

PART SEVEN

Chiropractic – Making a Difference

*Dr. Heather Dougherty-Harris D.C, F.I.C.P.A. and
Dr. Andrew K. Harris, D.C.*

For us, chiropractic is more than a profession – it is a way of life. Caring for and maintaining our spines and nervous systems help us balance, not merely juggle, the demands of everyday life.

To further support this, our lives include spirituality, positive mental attitude, loving relationships, proper sleep, fitness and nutrition. We feel this is the perfect recipe to allow our bodies to achieve and maintain wellness.

We define wellness as the state when the body, mind and spirit are all functioning at 100 percent capacity. We consider anything below 100 percent as unhealthy or illness.

Chiropractic is the cornerstone to maintaining the health of the nervous system through spinal adjustments. This is why we acknowledge chiropractic as the backbone of wellness!

We believe innate intelligence, which is the wisdom and ability to heal, resides in each one of us. Chiropractic care is founded on innate intelligence.

We practice this belief. It is reflected in our lifestyle both at our office and home. We share it with our children, friends, families and colleagues. We strive to be role models for others.

The Beginning

Our first practice was located in a fitness center in Pennsylvania. We eventually bought and restructured the fitness center converting the gym into a wellness facility. It was called "Health and Fitness Connection" and provided an outlet for our patients to learn to better care for their bodies.

Both of us understood, from early ages, the importance of taking care of our bodies, minds and spirits. Before we were doctors, as young chiropractic patients, we learned the value of healthy nervous systems. We discovered adjustments were the key to maintaining our overall health.

Before Andy became a chiropractic doctor, he was an electrical engineer. Andy was always interested in sports and physical fitness. He played rugby in his spare time. Andy's rugby coach was a chiropractor.

When pain from an injury was causing Andy to possibly miss a championship game, he went to his coach for chiropractic treatment.

Andy was amazed, after just one adjustment, how much better he felt. He was able to play in the big championship game. This experience eventually led him to re-enter college, study to become a doctor of chiropractic and change careers.

Heather was on her own at age 17 in New York. She led a busy life as an aerobics instructor and a budding interior designer.

One day, she bent over the bathroom sink to brush her teeth and couldn't stand up again. Friends took her to a hospital emergency room. Heather wasn't sure she wanted to take the prescribed muscle-relaxants.

Luckily, another friend referred her to a chiropractor. With adjustments over a period of time, the chiropractic doctor helped restore Heather's health. The doctor taught her the importance of allowing her body time to heal itself. Heather learned the value of maintaining a healthy nervous system with spinal adjustments.

Our chiropractors told each of us we would make great chiropractors. This led us to college for chiropractic studies. We met during our schooling.

We train our office staff to share their experiences with our patients, their families and the community. We feel this is vital. We may be asking some of our patients to make positive lifestyle modifications or changes. It helps for our patients to have a support team that includes doctors and staff.

To make these enhancements, we realize our patients learn in different ways. We use various methods to help our patients including seminars, workshops, books, literature and other educational tools.

We listen closely. Sometimes, it's what patients don't say which can also help us determine care.

Stress-Related Health Challenges

Patients come into the office with enormous amounts of stress. Often, they don't realize the ways in which the body could negatively react to mental, chemical and physical stress or trauma. People may be living longer today, but could be experiencing lower qualities of life because nervous systems may not be functioning at optimal levels.

We teach our patients the first step to achieving wellness is attaining optimally functioning spines and nervous systems. Then, we guide them toward lifestyle changes that will cultivate wellness.

People are bombarded with commercials touting that health challenges can be solved with pills. Some healthcare professionals have placed the power of healing inside a pill or upon "simple or routine surgery."

In our quick-fix, fast-paced society, some people expect medications to solve health issues, and solve them quickly.

We believe it is important to listen to the body's inner wisdom, tap into its ability to heal and allow wellness to exist naturally. For those who are willing to make positive lifestyles modifications and allow sufficient time for the healing process, results could be amazing.

Wellness is not here one day and gone the next. The creation or destruction of wellness is a process over a period of time. Achieving wellness requires a cumulative course of action.

We see people transform from patients to teachers and role models, sharing their success stories. They bring friends and families to the office to have their spines checked. Leading by example, they begin teaching their children how to respect and take care of their health and bodies.

It's rewarding for us when we see changes affecting an entire family. We believe their experiences will reach an entire population. This is how we know we have done our jobs. And, how we know, today, we have made a difference.

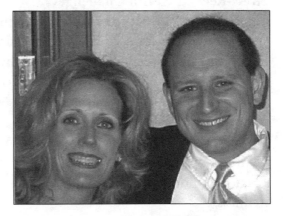

Dr. Heather Dougherty-Harris,
D.C, F.I.C.P.A. and
Dr. Andrew K. Harris, D.C.
Harris Family Chiropractic
Trappe, PA
610-489-8645

PART EIGHT

IMPROVING ATHLETIC ABILITY WITH CHIROPRACTIC CARE

~~~

By Dr. Thomas Kolenda, D.C.

While in the Air Force, I sustained a serious back injury. Over time, it intensified causing immense pain down both my legs. The pain was so severe that walking became difficult. My foot would drag causing me to trip occasionally.

Trying to find relief, I went to an orthopedic surgeon at the Veterans Hospital close to where I lived. The surgeon told me I would have to live with the pain. For a man in his twenties, this bleak prospect was extremely upsetting.

Soon after, a friend recommended I see a chiropractor he knew. With hopes of eliminating the pain, I made an appointment. The chiropractor discovered, instead of the normal 45% curvature of the spine, I had a 53% curvature. With too much curve, the bones were pressing down on the nerves causing pain.

After only three adjustments, the pain was greatly reduced; within six months, it was completely gone. I felt as if I had been given a new lease on life. I wanted to be a chiropractor and give the same gift of life to other people. Inspired by God, in 1995, I entered a chiropractic college.

Although I work with many different types of people and problems, the majority of my patients are talented athletes. Being an athlete myself, I understand the varying levels of trauma that can happen to the body. Some of my patients come to me with injuries to knees and feet caused by running and exercise or shoulder injuries from falling and landing wrong.

My wife, Vivian, has been an athlete much of her life. Prior to us getting together, in her twenties, she took up running which eventually caused severe knee pain. After a marathon at age 36, Vivian's knees worsened causing severe pain continuously. She was forced to stop running. The pain was only minimized. Vivian experienced great difficulty sitting for any length of time without stretching her legs.

Shunning surgery, she went on with life. She learned to "deal" with the pain believing this was how it would be. During this time, Vivian and I started dating; I began adjusting her. Within a short time, she was back to her level of optimal health.

Adjusted regularly, she experiences knee pain only on occasion and usually from something done out of the ordinary. With regular adjustments, not only does she live almost pain-free, she has also experienced a significant improvement with her allergies.

Winning Over Limitations

One particular patient came to me six weeks prior to running the London marathon. Suffering from severe shin splints, he was no longer able to train. This meant potentially giving up the marathon.

I placed him on an aggressive schedule of adjustments up until the time he left for London. After the marathon, he called to thank me. Not only did he finish, he qualified for the Boston Marathon with a finishing time of 3 hours and 28 minutes.

Typically, my athletic patients complain of limitations where their bodies are not able to function at full range. This might be a golfer not able to swing the club properly or a baseball player who has restricted use of the throwing arm. My goal is to bring patients to the place of their best ability.

A common problem with the body is subluxation where two

or more vertebrae are misaligned causing the nerves to be compressed. Once compressed, the nerves have difficulty communicating with the muscles, organs and tissues of the body. This could restrict the entire body from performing at its optimal level.

I believe educating patients on how to maintain optimal health is crucial. I can work with someone and bring him or her to their optimal level. Unless they maintain that level, chances are they will again experience problems.

After helping my patients reach their optimal levels of health and physical abilities, I encourage them to start wellness programs to keep their spines aligned. When the interference of subluxation is removed, the body could heal faster. A well-tuned athlete must be in his or her best physical condition and exercise to sustain an optimal performance level.

One of my patients illustrates this concept perfectly. This patient is a three-time national barefoot water-skiing champion. Although this young man is extremely talented, he took a bad spill in the water, injured his hip and twisted his knee. Through a course of corrective adjustments, he has continued skiing breaking even more records. He maintains his edge with wellness check-ups.

For the professional athlete, weekend warrior and non-athlete alike, chiropractic care can be beneficial to overall health and well-being.

Being Your Best

Unfortunately, many ailments do not present symptoms of physical pain so people assume they are healthy and do not need chiropractic care. What these people do not know is that approximately 10% of the nervous system's function has to do with pain sensation, while approximately 90% deals with the function of the body.

For example, with heart disease, the first symptom people feel could be a fatal heart attack.

Will chiropractic care prevent heart attacks? I am not sure, but I do know I want my heart working to the best of its ability. I want my spine to be in the best alignment possible so the nerves running from my spinal column to my heart do not have interference. Obviously, this same principle is applied to the entire spine and all of the organs and tissues of the body.

What Is Healing for You?

For some, "traditional medicine" means chemistry rather than biomechanics or movement of the body. People have become accustomed to seeing a medical doctor for pain. The result could be prescriptions that mask the pain, while the underlying causes of the pain may still not have been identified or treated.

We live in an "immediate gratification" world. Drugs may relieve pain immediately, although, at times, temporarily.

First-time patients may think with one or two chiropractic adjustments their problems will be gone. I remind my patients the body heals at its pace, not ours. Therefore, while one patient could have 100% relief within weeks, other patients might take longer.

In chiropractic care, it is important to keep the faith remembering the body is its own best physician. Everyone's bodies respond differently.

For example, if ten people are in the same room and one of them has the flu, not everyone will become sick. But, some will. This is because each person's immune system is functioning at a different level. If a person's immune system is not working at its optimal level, it cannot defend the body from all of the germs faced daily.

Since the immune system is tied directly to the nervous system, it only makes sense to keep the nervous system functioning at its highest level. This can be achieved through regular chiropractic care and reducing subluxations causing nerve interference.

If you were in a race — whether driving, riding or betting — wouldn't you want the best odds to win? Chiropractic care places the odds in your favor.

The body stores great knowledge. Removing pressure and opening the communication link between the spine and the nervous system can share this innate knowledge within the body so it can naturally heal. God has given me the gift of chiropractic care. I believe it is my responsibility, and one of my greatest joys, to share this gift with others.

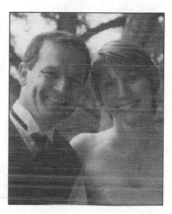

Dr. Thomas Kolenda, D.C.
and his wife Vivian.
Kolenda Chiropractic Clinic
Austin, TX
512-231-9002

Dr. Kolenda specializes in athletic performance with an emphasis on the knees, feet and hips.

PART NINE

CHIROPRACTIC... IT JUST MAKES SENSE

≈

By Dr. Joseph J. Frasco, D.C.

It was 1980, and I was in my third year at the University of Rhode Island contemplating what I would do with the rest of my life.

Unlike my brother, who was encouraged to enter the pre-med program at Villanova University and medical school at Tufts, I was an independent thinker and did not receive much direction from my parents.

It was during a weekend spent with my brother and his friends that I began to seriously explore my future. Acting on their suggestions, I looked into being a chiropractor. At that time, however, I didn't even know what a chiropractor did.

Later that same week, I found myself in the university's library looking up "chiropractic," only to find there was just one book on the subject. As it turned out, the book was written by a medical doctor making a case against chiropractic care.

This Intrigued Me More

A few days later, I went to the admissions office to ask about chiropractic colleges. In an effort to assist me, the receptionist began looking through the files to find the information I needed. She came up with nothing.

There was information on pre-med, pre-dentistry and even

pre-veterinarian, but nothing on chiropractic. I thanked her for her help. I started to leave when she suggested we look in the phonebook. She then called and made arrangements for me to see chiropractors.

Looking back, I can't remember her name. I just know that was the turning point for my life and my entire future.

Local Chiropractor

I clearly remember walking up to his farmhouse which doubled as his home and office, ringing the doorbell and meeting the doctor. He was friendly and interested in me, because I was interested in chiropractic.

During that day, he spent time explaining chiropractic care, showing me diagrams of the human spinal column and detailing how the nervous system is the master of the entire body. He showed me how the nervous system is housed in and protected by the spinal column. He talked about how displacements of the spinal vertebrae could interfere with communications between the brain and the body. He said this could lead to terrible health problems.

It made sense to me, and I was hooked.

I quickly volunteered to help him once a week and began that Friday.

I showed up to find him finishing his breakfast and preparing to see patients. The wood stove gave the home/office a cozy feel. Not long after I arrived, the waiting room filled with patients.

There were three examination rooms and no receptionist. Patients continuously told me stories of how conventional medical treatment had failed them. They talked about how their health had been restored and improved through chiropractic care.

I began telling everyone I knew I was going to be a chiropractor.

My decision was met with mixed reactions including, "A what?" I was often asked: "What do chiropractors do?" and "Is chiropractic care for real?"

I did not let this sway me. I knew chiropractic care worked. I had seen firsthand.

Admittedly, I did find their responses intriguing. I was also intrigued by the fact there is an entire profession licensed by the United States Government in all 50 states, with 16 accredited colleges, and no one seemed to know much about it.

The chiropractic profession represents the largest drugless healthcare profession in the world. Chiropractic care promotes wellness and restoration of health without drugs and surgery.

What if a majority of the American population opted for chiropractic care? Could the need for expensive drugs and medical procedures be reduced? I see more and more people choosing chiropractic care every year.

Chiropractic care has given me a unique perspective on health; how we loose it and how it can be restored. I have come to respect the power of the human mind to heal and rejuvenate.

I understand the positive results produced by chiropractic care and the natural approach to health restoration. The healing ability inside your body is there for you. Try chiropractic, which is what millions of people worldwide have chosen. Respect your body. Choose to work with a chiropractor; show yourself and your family a natural, healing way to health and wellness!

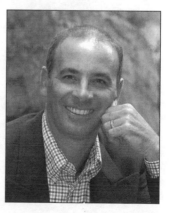

Dr. Joseph J. Frasco
Frasco Chiropractic
New Providence, NJ
908-771-0707

CHAPTER SIX

HOW TO PROTECT
YOUR FAMILY

PART ONE

THE INCREDIBLE HUMAN BODY

≈

By Dr. Dan Larsen, D.C.

As a doctor of chiropractic, I have a deep respect and admiration for the human body's amazing ability to heal itself without the use of surgery or medication. I believe the best pharmacy in the world can be found inside each and every one of us. Chiropractic is the natural key that unlocks our body's healing power, giving it the opportunity to function at its best.

The roots of chiropractic care can be traced all the way back to ancient China and Greece. In the United States, chiropractic first started gaining popularity in the late nineteenth century in Iowa.

Several generations from my mother's side of the family were farmers and used to rely on chiropractors for all their health care needs. Whenever someone would get sick, he or she would get adjusted. I learned the benefits of chiropractic care very early in life and feel a strong personal connection to this healing art.

Several members of my immediate family, including my father, are mainstream medical professionals. There was never a doubt in my mind that I wanted to practice chiropractic's non-invasive and drug-free healing.

While mainstream medicine in this country is outstanding for crisis and emergency situations, a holistic approach, in my opinion, could work much better for preventive care and overall wellness.

Chiropractors consider every patient as an integrated being and get to the root cause of the problem. I believe no other profession focuses on the intimate relationship of the body and its nervous system to help achieve optimal health.

It is my belief, society has programmed many people from early on to ignore our bodies' demands. Why not listen to our bodies? How about closely examining every symptom as a possible indicator of a more serious condition?

In my opinion, Americans take too many prescription and non-prescription drugs as the way to eliminate aches and pains. Could these drugs be causing damage?

I believe, as a nation, we are currently experiencing a real "wellnesscare revolution." More and more people are opting for natural and non-invasive techniques for better quality of life.

During my seven years in practice, I have been seeing patients for neck and back pains, headaches and many other conditions. They trust my chiropractic judgment and professional expertise. Having the opportunity to help and provide chiropractic care is the most gratifying experience in the world.

Phases of Care

In my office, patients go through three phases of care. The first is the initial, intensive phase where the goal is to alleviate pain. The second is where the spine is corrected. The third is the wellness phase. I believe this phase to be most important. It is during this phase that the spine and nervous system are kept optimally running.

It is important for new patients to realize most conditions have been building over time and will be impossible to fix overnight. When you take a pill, it could fool the nerves into thinking everything is fine. It provides immediate, but short-term, relief. The new generation of chiropractic patients understands real healing requires time.

The first and most important step in chiropractic care is the adjustment of the nervous system. When patients start feeling better, they are usually more motivated to keep improving their levels of wellness and fitness through moderate exercise and good nutrition. All my patients learn basic nutritional requirements and receive recommendations regarding various stretching techniques and exercises most appropriate for their particular condition.

Education is paramount, as it is crucial for chiropractic patients to better understand and appreciate their own bodies. An increasing number of people are becoming more educated about chiropractic healing even prior to their first visits to chiropractors.

In response to the growing interest in natural healing and holistic health, I offer regular workshops and give materials to help educate people about the benefits of a healthy spine through chiropractic care. I keep workshops interactive and open a real dialogue to make sure attendees participate and share experiences.

More Than Just One Thing

Some patients may come into a chiropractor's office with a thought that one particular habit was responsible for all their health problems, which of course, is not the case. In fact, it is usually never *one* particular thing. Rather, it is usually a combination of several factors such as stress, lack of exercise and improper diet causing nerve interference and health problems.

New patients are often under the impression their symptoms have been caused by a few extra hours of garden work or a vigorous exercise session. The reality is that the events they hold responsible have usually triggered pre-existing conditions resulting from years of unhealthy lifestyles.

A patient, who turns to a chiropractor for the first time with a particular health problem, could quickly realize the numerous benefits of this non-invasive approach to healing. He or she is eager to share this newly acquired knowledge with loved ones. Chiropractic healing could quickly become a "family affair."

Could it be we are seeing an increase in the number of first-time patients who come to firmly believe chiropractic care is the best care for their children?

Chiropractic care can start long before the baby is born. It could be an essential choice in overall prenatal care. Can you see how a woman, who found comfort through chiropractic care during her pregnancy, could desire to bring her child to her chiropractor's office for a subluxation check several weeks or even days after birth?

A chiropractor's job is more than aligning the spine to provide immediate and short-term relief from back, neck or shoulder pain. Prevention is an integral part of chiropractic healing. There is a significant difference between relief care and corrective care.

In recovery from aches and pains, as well as, achieving overall health and wellness, chiropractic care has proven its effectiveness for many of my patients. There is no greater reward than observing true miracles taking place in my office as people reap the benefits of chiropractic and experience positive changes in their health and overall quality of life.

One of my patients, who suffered multiple injuries from two serious car crashes, came to me when she felt she had "nothing to lose." This is what she had to say after several months of chiropractic care:

"Thanks to Dr. Dan Larsen and his staff, my life is better than I had hoped for myself.

"After five years of treatments under my car insurance plan, I was told I was as good as I would ever get. I still had neck, shoulder, elbow, upper back, lower back, hip and knee problems. I could barely get around unassisted. I was trying to keep as mobile as possible by going to the gym and exercising.

"When I was finally referred to Dr. Larsen, I was skeptical

because of my past experiences with medical professionals. I went anyway because there was nothing to lose.

"Dr. Dan did initial exams including X-rays. He listened to a long list of illnesses. Along with the chiropractic care, I also received massage therapy and physical therapy in his office. Dr. Dan was always positive and encouraging, helping me make it through the little setbacks along the road to recovery.

"Through the care of Dr. Dan and his support staff, I am improving. I've learned to live again with less pain medication, get around much better and pace myself so I could do more. A great big thanks to Dr. Dan Larsen and his staff."

We are born with tremendous physical, emotional and intellectual potential. The goal is to activate, access and actualize this potential while achieving and maintaining optimal health.

Wellness could be described as a condition that helps us feel, look and do our best. The pursuit of wellness often has a profound effect on my patients' minds and emotional well-being. It inspires them to discover and explore their capacity for success and happiness in everyday life.

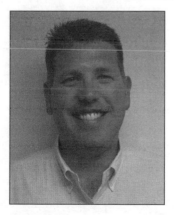

Dr. Dan Larsen, D.C.
Larsen Chiropractic & Wellness Center
Lakewood, CO
303-934-2116

PART TWO

THE PERMANENT SOLUTION

~~~

By Dr. Michael J. Smith, D.C.

The Greek poet Heraclitus once said: "It is impossible to point to the same spot in the river twice because the water is always flowing." Like a river, our life is constantly changing and sometimes overflowing with new challenges.

When faced with stressful situations and difficult choices, it is crucial to maintain a sense of inner balance and harmony in the midst of outer activity. By focusing attention on achieving optimal functioning of our bodies, we can revitalize our minds and seek our true nature as spiritual beings having a human experience.

Since late 1800's, chiropractic remains a classic holistic approach to achieving and maintaining wellness by correcting subluxations of the spine. As a result of the growing public awareness about chiropractic, millions of people have experienced profound changes in the qualities of their lives. This has been accomplished through the art, science and philosophy of locating and correcting spinal subluxations.

As a doctor of chiropractic, I define wellness as an optimal state of physical, emotional and spiritual well-being achieved through a balanced diet, proper exercise and spinal health.

Getting Started

First-time patients generally turn to a chiropractor when they experience symptoms they associate with specific, recent events.

There can be other underlying causes of their health problems. Ergonomic strains at work, stressful relationships, unhealthy lifestyles or recent traumas could also be to blame. Prolonged stress could create emotional and physical changes damaging the body, decreasing energy and causing fatigue.

Experienced chiropractors see beyond symptoms. They consider each patient as an integrated individual with dreams, desires and aspirations, as well as, problems, challenges and fears. However, I keep in mind that it was the symptoms which brought the patient into the office.

Patients usually have to make decisions as to how much time, money and energy they are able to devote to chiropractic care. It is imperative to provide patients the most complete and accurate information possible. Taking care of symptoms is an important first phase. This could allow doors to open to a more comprehensive healthy lifestyle through chiropractic.

I feel communication is the secret for a successful doctor-patient relationship. My patients and I work as a team. Our first appointment together serves as an introduction. With the opportunity to ask questions, I am able to learn more about the patient's health challenges. As his or her doctor, I am interested in lifestyle, work demands, recreational activities, diet and other factors that could contribute to the current level of health and wellness. In addition to listening to my patient very carefully, I perform a complete physical exam including appropriate x-rays.

Doctors of chiropractic were among the first healthcare professionals to realize the diagnostic benefits of x-rays. B.J. Palmer, known as the developer of chiropractic, became one of the first health educators in the world to include the new x-ray imagining technology, or as he called it "spinography," as part of Palmer College of Chiropractic curriculum in 1910. X-rays had been discovered in France in 1895, which is the same year chiropractic was born.

X-rays help diagnose problems, as well as document a patient's progress. With the advancement of high-speed film and limited exposure, in my opinion, the minimal amount of radiation used is far outweighed by the useful information gained by actually seeing the patient's spine.

I take front, back and side-view x-rays of each patient. I draw a black line on the x-ray showing the patient where his or her spine should be. Then, a red line is drawn showing the current position of his or her spine. The ultimate goal is to get the red line on top of the black line, or to return his or her spine to a normal, healthy position.

After putting all the diagnostic information together, I sit with each patient and explain my findings and my recommendations for care. I try to include a patient's spouse, significant other or a family member. This helps to make the patient's family aware of the situation and provide support and understanding during the healing process.

I feel the most profound way to improve and maintain health is through long-term chiropractic care. Some patients first start with a specific health concern. One person may want help with his or her back pain. Another may be trying to rid frequent headaches. A third may be seeking advice on improving posture.

Each of these needs is important in its own right. The positive results and relief could be the beginning of a patient integrating chiropractic into a health plan for overall wellness.

Chiropractic Empowerment

Part of my job is to help people learn to appreciate and properly care for their bodies. Ultimately, the choice is up to the individual.

I empower patients to make choices based on their unique needs and circumstances. Let's say a person's initial priority is to simply get out of pain and "to patch things up." With relief and results, he or she could choose a regular schedule of subluxation correction and wellnesscare.

Some people could feel skeptical, or even fearful, when they first start chiropractic care. I explain procedures and what may be felt or heard during an adjustment to help alleviate fears.

One may hear a "cracking sound" during the adjustment. This is the release of nitrogen and other gases from the joint capsule. It sounds similar to when one "cracks" his or her knuckles.

I treat patients with respect and compassion. I encourage them to take interest in their own bodies, health and well-being by asking questions. I provide answers in a way to serve them best.

The most exhilarating experiences in the world are to help people reclaim their health and quality of life and tap into their inner reservoirs of unlimited energy, creativity and vitality.

Like an artist creating a great piece of art, I feel inspired and passionate about strengthening people's spines. By performing adjustments to correct spines from subluxation and improper positioning, my goal is to improve the health and well-being of all my patients.

A doctor, by definition, is someone who both provides care and education. It is not surprising that patients regard their chiropractors as life mentors.

I am fascinated when I see long-term patients offering support and reassurance to new patients. Then, the new patients offer advice and encouragement to the next group of new patients. This allows the circle of health and healing to grow and continue.

You Are in Control

The positive effects of chiropractic are indisputable. The extent to which you choose to benefit from chiropractic care is ultimately up to you. You are responsible for the quality of your health and well-being. More and more patients are choosing chiropractic as their permanent solution for a lifetime of wellness. You can influence your health and well-being through the choices you make.

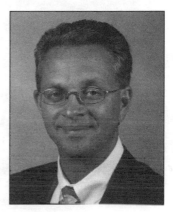

Dr. Michael J. Smith, D.C.
Waterside Chiropractic
Santa Rosa Beach, FL
850-622-0062

PART THREE

THE DOCTOR WITHIN:
THE EFFECTS OF CORRECTIVE CHIROPRACTIC ON THE IMMUNE SYSTEM

❧

By Dr. Bruce Wong, D.C.

In my practice, as well as my personal life, I've been witness to a phenomenon that never fails to amaze me. It seems that the more committed a patient becomes to their corrective chiropractic care, the less often they experience colds, flu or any type of illness.

Since becoming a corrective chiropractic patient myself in 1983, I have yet to miss a single day of work because of sickness. I've also got the stamina needed to provide care to a large number of patients each week, with enough energy left over to keep up with a brand new, baby daughter.

I have not stumbled upon some miracle cure or fountain of youth. In fact, there is nothing mysterious about this ability to fight disease. What I am describing is nothing more than the body's natural abilities to regenerate and repair, working at peak efficiency through chiropractic adjustments.

To quote D.D. Palmer, the founder of chiropractic, "to adjust subluxation is to advance mankind, step up his efficiency, increase his ability and make him more natural and more at peace."

Your body is made up of trillions of cells constantly regenerating. This regeneration is accomplished through messages sent from your brain to each organ through your spinal column.

These communications direct the regeneration of your liver, new red blood cells and epidermal skin layer.

This type of regeneration helps you stay healthy and alive.

Of course, a few of those trillion cells are bound to be weakened or abnormal in some way. When they are, trouble could follow. The abnormal cells, such as cancer cells, can begin to congregate and reproduce in a particular area of the body.

Fortunately, your immune system has you covered. Working like a microscopic Pac-Man®, cells from your immune system hunt down and devour the troublemakers, stopping health problems before irreversible damage is done.

It is a perfect relationship between your brain and nerves when messages to regenerate and repair can freely travel to every cell in your body.

Communication Cut

What would happen if the nerve to the liver was cut off by subluxation? The liver could begin to lose its function. It could not recreate or repair itself.

With spinal misalignment, otherwise called subluxation, there is a reduction in nerve flow. Subluxation could block or significantly reduce the signals sent from the brain down the spinal column to the liver. Years may pass before a person even noticed a problem or symptom. This organ could slowly and systematically be destroyed.

Unfortunately, this sort of "hidden" disease could be all too common. In a July 3, 2002, CBS News article, according to a cancer study, "Autopsy evidence has shown that 36 percent of white men and 28 percent of black men turned out to have had prostate cancer when they get an autopsy after dying of something else."

No one, not the doctors, not even the patients, knew the cancer was present until after death.

If cancer could be harbored without knowing it, imagine

how easy it might be to overlook heart disease, which could develop for decades without symptoms, or to believe you "just have indigestion" instead of a bleeding ulcer.

Now, imagine how miraculous it would be if health challenges could be prevented in their earliest stages.

This could be possible when you fully employ your body's innate ability to heal. With the adjustments of corrective chiropractic, you can remove nerve interference. This could allow the nerve system to send the full strength of its healing and regenerating powers to the liver, the heart or anywhere else it is needed.

Your nerve system is the channel for all healing and regeneration communications in the human body. You could be allowing for an internal therapeutic healing to take place.

I believe, on its own, the body will concentrate on the most significant health problem first, even if it's not the first problem that brought you to the chiropractor. Your body will ask for patience to wait for the completion of healing.

If my practice has taught me anything, it's that God's intelligence is always far greater than our own. I believe what some people need is not another medication, but the freedom to heal.

How can one employ a natural boost to his or her immune system? Education is the key. Learn about the different types of chiropractic (symptomatic vs. corrective). Then have a complete set of diagnostic examinations and x-rays completed by your chiropractic doctor. These findings could diagnose your unique subluxations and pinpoint exactly which nerves and systems are experiencing interference.

Wellness is not a destination point, rather a lifelong journey. The stresses of every day life could constantly cause subluxations. Nerve interference will need to be continuously addressed to maintain wellness.

To keep your nerve flow in optimal health, learn to practice chiropractic principles on a daily basis. Become as dedicated to your nervous system as you are to your daily dental practices.

No one would brush and floss for thirty years, only to stop one day and never brush again for the next thirty years! The damage to your teeth would be unimaginable.

It is exactly the same way with corrective chiropractic. Only by identifying, addressing and correcting physical, mental and chemical stressors will you be able to achieve maximum health potential in mind, body and spirit.

The definition of insanity is to keep trying the same thing, but expecting different results.

If the big, fluffy pillow you've been sleeping on is the cause of your spinal misalignments, you'll have to make a change. If you know how to eat right, but don't do it, you have to make a change or you could compromise your health in many ways.

Regardless of what everyone else is doing, accept the fact healing does not come from the outside. The only place you'll ever find healing is within your own body, your own mind and your own spirit. Embrace this and you'll find your new life could be far greater.

Dr. Bruce Wong, D.C.
Chiropractic USA
Honolulu, HI
808-593-2807

PART FOUR

HOW TO LIVE AN OUTRAGEOUSLY HEALTHY LIFE

By Dr. Daniel J. Hill, D.C.

It is possible to live a balanced life so you can be all you are meant to be and live outrageously healthy!

I have an acronym that spells out exactly what you have to do to get there. It is: GET PASSION. When practiced in a gentle but persistent fashion, you could experience marvelous and healthy results. Taking each letter, it works like this:

God/Spirituality

It is generally agreed individuals are comprised of mind, body and spirit. In general, we are very good at using our intellect to find solutions to all sorts of problems. We are becoming more aware of our health as people begin to take exercise and nutrition seriously. Often overlooked, however, is the spirit. And, if it isn't overlooked, it's either minimized or intellectualized.

We need to exercise our spiritual muscles, just as we exercise the muscles of the body. The goal is connecting with God or a Higher Power or the Universal Source (what you call It doesn't matter) so through this spiritual energy we can discover our precise purposes here and learn to actualize them.

I find the most direct method of accessing this knowledge and power is through prayer and meditation. Exactly what form you use is up to your desires. When prayer and meditation is practiced on a regular basis, you'll soon discover benefits of peace and knowledge.

Education

We live with an abundance of information about health.

We're bombarded by advertisements touting various pills for all sorts of real and imagined problems. Every day, it seems, a new study is released that opposes a study released last week. Combine this with the incredible amount of good, bad and indifferent information found on the Internet. The only real solution is to either become a health professional yourself or to work closely with one.

I recognize a major part of my role as a chiropractor is to coach people through the maze of health information. Working together, we sort through what they've heard, what they believe and their goals. We design a program including all aspects of their health from food through chiropractic adjustments. Equipped with accurate information, members of my community are able to take charge of their health in new and positive ways.

Time Out

Whenever I hear someone complain life has become so busy they hardly have time to think, I tell them, "You need time-out!" A time-out gives your body, mind and spirit a chance to rest, heal and regenerate.

You need a time-out when you lose your focus and your passion or when you find yourself impatient and feeling like snapping at people.

Vacations are obvious time-outs. I believe everyone should have at least four weeks a year away from his or her job. If a week or two is all you can manage, by all means take it.

Micro-vacations, or three-day weekends, are great time-outs. You'll come back refreshed and more productive. Even a few moments of quiet time inside or outside your office can do wonders when you do this consistently.

Powerful Posture

It's absolutely amazing how posture could affect your health, your mind and your spirit. Think of it this way. Your posture is the window to your spine. Your energy flows through your spine.

When a spine is aligned properly, energy is allowed to flow freely. When it is out of alignment, energy could be slowed or blocked. It's my job as a chiropractor to adjust and align your spine so your energy flows without restraint.

How often a person needs an adjustment depends on many factors. Ideally, each person starts with a complete structural-neurological checkup. This will reveal any problems and point the way toward proper care.

In my opinion, it is a good idea for children to have a structural-neurological checkup as well. Many of the problems chiropractors address actually start when patients are youngsters. The sooner detected, the quicker problems can be corrected potentially preventing future agony and ill health.

Aerobic Exercise and Breath

Simply put, if the cells in your body don't get enough oxygen, they will mutate or die. The oxygen they need comes with your breath. Aerobic exercise is important. It strengthens your whole cardio-vascular system. It is also an excellent way to engage in truly deep breathing. After checking with your chiropractor, a goal could be 15 to 20 minutes of aerobic activity at least two or three times a week.

Stretch

Stretching is magic. It opens you up, encourages deeper breathing, relieves tired muscles (and protects them against injury) and can act as an effective mini time-out.

A simple goal could be five to ten minutes of stretching at least five days a week. You can incorporate it into your prayer and meditation time with good results.

I arrive to my office an hour before anyone else. I pray, meditate and stretch. This is my sacred time to center and focus.

Remember micro-stretch breaks, particularly if you're sitting or standing for long periods of time. Quick stretch breaks every hour will make you feel better and increase your productivity as well.

Sleep

A good night's sleep, in my opinion, is a must for outrageous health. Sleep can allow bodies to heal and deeply recharge. Dreams could help relieve stress.

While asleep, a body feels only minimal affects from gravity. Gravity is constantly pulling on us. Over time, gravity could cause breakdown of the body. Give your body a break; get enough sleep.

How much is enough? Sleep requirements and patterns are highly individual. They change over time. As a general rule, however, people could use between six and eight hours of sleep each night.

Invest in Supplements and Nutrition

It's almost impossible to find the vitamins and minerals you need from food alone. Much of our soil is depleted or laden with chemicals. Many foods are processed. Busy lives can mean not making the time to eat properly.

Good vitamin and mineral supplementation could be an answer. I like liquid supplements for several reasons. Given to children, we're not teaching them pills are the answer. The body tends to absorb the vitamins and minerals in the liquid more quickly and completely than in many pill forms.

Water is another important factor in nutrition – lots of it. I personally use this formula: Body weight divided by two; change pounds to ounces. That's how much water I recommend a person drink daily. If you weighed 200 pounds, divide by 2 and you have 100 pounds. Change the pounds to ounces. In this scenario, you'd need 100 ounces of water daily.

Outrageous Victories

Give yourself credit. Celebrate your successes and victories. Not just the big ones, like a promotion or a winning golf score, but the little ones too. Small victories count like smiling at someone who is discouraged or being polite to the impolite lane-changer in traffic.

Why Do This?

You deserve credit. You deserve celebrations that help bring your view of yourself into real balance. We're all pretty hard on ourselves, feeling we should have done more or done it better. In truth, we're all doing the very best we can in each individual moment. So celebrate and the more outrageously the better.

Keep track of your victories in a journal. Take a moment or two at the end of the day and write them down. Reread your journal on those days you feel most discouraged. You'll be delighted and amazed at how much better you feel.

Nuclear Power

The human body is amazing. In emergency situations, it can go a month without food and days without water. But, as soon as the nerve flow stops, we die.

Our health depends on energy flow. This runs from brain through spine to all nerves, muscles, organs and back again.

Subluxations or misalignments of the spine prevent us from achieving our God given potential. Adjustments connect us to our healing source, our God source.

Are you connected?

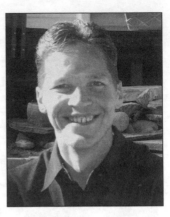

Dr. Daniel J. Hill, D.C., CCEP
Cottonwood Chiropractic
Parker, CO
303-840-3535
www.practicewellness.com

Dr. Hill's practice specializes in family wellness, preventative health and sports chiropractic care. Dr. Hill was hired as one of two official team chiropractors for the two-time NFL champion Denver Broncos when the team integrated chiropractic into their full-time fitness regime. Dr. Hill provided chiropractic care to the players at least twice per week during the regular and off seasons.

PART FIVE

A QUESTION OF FAITH (AND SCIENCE)

By Dr. Matthew Stockstad, D.C.

I have chosen to follow what many people see as two different paths. One is the path of faith. The other is the path of science.

Faith is a mysterious force; it cannot be seen or measured in scientific terms.

Science focuses on the tangible and measurable. Science seems to exclude faith.

Since I was a child, I wanted a way to bring faith and science together. This desire has formed the basis of my search and become the foundation of my life.

Faith was my first search. I longed for proof that a divine power was active and living within our world. In college, I earned a Masters Degree in Divinity and gained a perspective in which God creates, maintains and sustains His creation.

This increased my understanding and faith in the ongoing process of life. We can witness this higher power in our daily events. We may take God-like experiences for granted, such as cuts healing or people walking, because they naturally occur.

When they do not occur, we are shaken and seek other means to have the power restored. We could find ourselves going to see a doctor or kneeling to pray.

While I was doing internship as a chaplain in Dorothea Dix Psychiatric Hospital in Raleigh, N.C., I found my answer.

There I observed both science and faith at work. While medicine offered much in the treatment of a patient's physical condition, it fell short in addressing the mental anguish and despair people suffered over the deterioration of their health.

Medicine alone, it seemed, could not provide them with the strength or will to heal. This came from another source. This brought me full circle to confirming God could be the origin and maintainer of our health. Ultimately, I saw the patients find health and healing within themselves. If a person does not have the faith and will to live, healing is undermined.

Now, also as a doctor of chiropractic, the question is how can we lead patients from illness to health?

The science of chiropractic looks at the body as a structural entity that can be adjusted with very predictable outcomes.

It is much like looking at an automobile with a front tire turned out a mere 15 degrees. If the tire is fairly new, we may not be able to see the signs of the degenerative changes. But with time, we know the inside of the tire will wear faster. We also know the gas mileage could be less. This car will pull slightly to one side. The life of the engine could be reduced due to the increased stress.

Science in Need of Faith

As a hospital chaplain my heart was touched with words of despair. Yet more so, I was touched with words of faith uttered by people facing life and death situations.

As a chiropractor, in my office I would sit face-to-face with patients who asked me to label their diseases. In my early practice, it was easy to give disease a name and act as if the disease was bigger than the patient.

At times, it seemed, the patient became disease. Their names changes from John or Mary to cancer. I have seen all too often a person's disease named and then watch that person die. Hope is often the first thing lost. The will to live frequently follows, until finally death of the body occurs.

I have also seen, in the face of being told the name of a disease, a person laugh at the words knowing they were so much bigger than the words themselves. I share this message often with my patients.

What are the boundaries defining our lives and giving us power over our own experiences of sickness and disease?

I let my patients know they are not alone in the health crisis they could be experiencing. I ask them to remove hopeless thoughts from their minds and draw from a power much bigger than us.

I have the pleasure of seeing the power of faith being restored in my patients' lives through science and chiropractic. Many could look upon what I do as healing. In my practice, the chiropractic adjustment releases and ignites the healer residing within each patient.

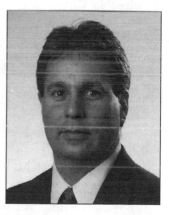

Dr. Matthew Stockstad, D.C.
Stockstad Family Chiropractic
Asheville, NC
828-299-4555

PART SIX

HEALING
TAKES TIME

❧

By Dr. Julie Peterson, D.C.

All processes require time including the process of you!

Even with immediate change, whether with the first adjustment, the first week of a diet or the first week of running, lasting results take time.

We have become accustom to expect quick fixes. Is relief really only a pill or a swallow away?

I question an outside-in health philosophy. I don't believe there is a pill, potion or lotion with better odds of helping you than you deciding to help yourself from the inside-out.

Mystery of Health

Isn't it a mystery how true health takes time to achieve? And, can be lost so quickly?

Follow me here. Imagine committing to exercise for 10 years. Then, you suddenly stop. The benefits of 10 years of fitness could be lost in a matter of weeks.

The same may be true for most events that contribute to our health such as brushing your teeth, your spiritual practice, working out, lifetime weekly chiropractic adjustments and eating clean food from health food stores.

Illness Takes Time

A loss of health does not happen overnight, even though it may seem to have snuck up on you. A loss of health could be a result of subluxations and bad habits accumulating over time.

We often wish healing would be immediate and precisely the way we want it.

I believe the body has innate intelligence that knows the right way and the right time. Healing may not happen in a straight line. Sometimes we may even seem to worsen before we get better. While healing, a body might plateau at a holding place appearing to be stagnant. When we do the right things long enough, the end results can be fairly predictable.

A gardener planting bulbs and seeds carefully tends and prepares the soil for the best results. Does the gardener expect to see fully grown plants with flowers ready to cut the next day? Sound ridiculous?

Why is it we expect our bodies to transform after one adjustment? We could choose to trust the natural healing process of our bodies just as the gardener will trust the ability of the bulb to transform into a spectacular plant.

Bodies heal from the inside-out. I believe for true health to happen, change must first occur on a cellular level.

New, improved cells start to join together to form tissues. Tissues join together and form organs. Organs with similar purpose are called systems such as your digestive system or reproductive system. Systems unite to form the most amazing thing…you.

Your brain is the conductor of this ultimate organization. Direction flows down the spinal cord out to each cell, tissue, organ and system. All have a direct line of communication to the brain. This creates organization and coordination resulting in harmony within the body. This unity can be disrupted when subluxation or nerve interference is present.

This organization and coordination is why it may take time for whole systems to be reworked.

Waiting until something is "broken" or not working properly requires time for your body to create the symptom. Once a symptom shows up in your body, it could take a lot of time to heal both the symptom and the cause.

If we experienced a terrible cut, we could watch the cut's progress from an open sore to red, inflamed scab to pale white scar to new tissue.

While we heal inside-out, we see only the END result, not the inner healing.

During true healing, the body will sometimes feel worse before it gets better. Have you experienced this? Towards the end of a cold or flu, your fever may increase and you feel really miserable. But the next day, it's over and you feel the change.

I believe the greatest doctor lives inside of you. I feel there is no pill, potion or lotion with greater ability to fix you than you. True health comes from within and by doing the right things long enough. Cell-by-cell your true potential could become maximized. I believe we must put enough time into healing to first repair, then restore and finally replenish our bodies.

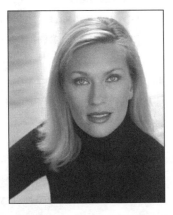

Be patient with your body. Put your time in consistently and thoughtfully healing until each part of you flourishes.

Healing takes time!

Dr. Julie Peterson, D.C.
Harbor View Chiropractic
Charleston, SC
843-795-3456

Dr. Julie Peterson practices in Charleston, South Carolina. She focuses on family care. Half of her practice members are children. She is a National Spokesperson for American Mensa. Since 2001, Julie has hosted her nationally syndicated radio show, *Health Watch*, with CNN Radio.

PART SEVEN

GETTING A WELLNESS CHIROPRACTOR ON YOUR HEALTH TEAM

By Dr. Amy Michelle Willcockson, D.C.

In high school, while competing in cheerleading and dance, I suffered an injury that threatened to end my athletic career. Instead of taking me to a medical doctor, my father took me to see his chiropractor. This is where my passion for chiropractic began.

Immediately after treatment, I felt better and was able to continue participating in cheerleading and dance. The result of that single visit sparked my interest and began my own wellness journey.

The Wellness Chiropractor

Wellness chiropractors will put your quality of life first above all else. They will challenge the way you currently view health care and engage you in an extremely powerful mindset. This could ultimately lead you to adopt new ways of thinking about your health. They will reveal why it is vital to maintain a healthy balance of mind, body and spirit, as well as, teach you how to achieve a successful "wellness attitude."

*"Each patient carries his own doctor inside him. They come to us
not knowing that truth. We are at our best when we give the
doctor who resides within each patient a chance to work."*
– Albert Schweitzer, M.D.

Your body heals itself. This philosophy invites you to trust your own natural healing abilities.

A proactive approach to your health includes good nutrition, spinal health care, proper exercise and stress management. For some of us, this shift to prevention thinking comes naturally. For others, learning a new approach to health may require conscious effort. A wellness attitude will be a positive and rewarding decision that will improve the quality of you and your family's lives forever.

*"While other professions are concerned with changing the
environment to suit the weakened body, chiropractic is concerned
with strengthening the body to suit the environment."*
– B.J. Palmer, D.C.

Your wellness attitude begins with a strong healthy spine which is the foundation of a wellness-oriented lifestyle. Dysfunctional areas in your spine are called vertebral subluxations. These subluxations could interfere with your brain's ability to heal and regulate functions.

Wellness chiropractors use gentle, effective adjustments to correct these subluxations. Once corrected, continued adjustments maintain the higher level of health associated with an optimally functioning spine and nervous system.

Maintaining this higher level of health requires that you take care of your spine just as you would anything else. You change the oil in your car to maximize its performance and brush your teeth to keep them from decaying. Wellness chiropractors will provide a maintenance program for your spine based on the following facts:

1. Your spine should be regularly maintained from birth throughout your entire life. Why? Because you cannot escape the effects of gravity, avoid accidents or prevent many impacts common to daily life.

2. Vertebral subluxation cannot be felt. Subluxations could exist in your body for years prior to detection. When your spine is misaligned, the nervous system could experience interference communicating with the rest of the body. Although this breakdown in communication could affect the body's ability to heal, you feel nothing out of the ordinary.

3. The condition could become worse if left undetected and uncorrected. Subluxated spines can be weak and could develop deformities leading to degenerative problems, such as herniated discs and arthritis.

In my experience, many symptoms people suffer are simply the effects of subluxation. Backaches, headaches, neck pain, indigestion, ear infections and allergies are common, but they are not normal. Each time you experience an ache or pain, your body could be communicating a malfunction.

If caught in time, wellness chiropractors could relieve common symptoms, as well as, correct the underlying cause. The opportunity to be free of aches and pains enables you to embrace your wellness attitude.

In order to maintain optimal spinal health and a strong wellness attitude, I feel it is essential to schedule regular chiropractic check-ups. These check-ups should have the same, if not greater, level of importance as any dental or eye examination.

A wellness chiropractor provides a thorough consultation and complete examination to determine the frequency of care necessary to correct any subluxations found in your spine. Once corrected, it is important to establish a maintenance schedule to prevent subluxation from reoccurring and sustain your higher level of health.

> *"Chiropractors adjust subluxations, relieving pressure*
> *from the nerves so that they can perform their*
> *functions in a normal matter."*
> – B.J. Palmer, D.C.

A wellness chiropractor's primary purpose is the correction of nerve interference caused by subluxation. This interference could weaken your immune system, promote sickness and disease and prevent you from expressing your God given potential.

Chiropractic is a natural method of internal healing, free of drugs and invasive surgeries. Over 60,000 chiropractors care for their communities worldwide with more than 25 million people utilizing chiropractic each year.

As a member of the chiropractic community, I work with my colleagues to heighten awareness of subluxation making it a household word. We do this by providing educational workshops at businesses, senior centers, schools, as well as, spinal screenings at health fairs and community events.

Your wellness chiropractor will encourage you to share your wellness attitude and understanding of subluxation with your friends, family, co-workers and any one else who desires to live life to its fullest.

The future of our world depends on the health of the next generation. Children are our future. They need the tools to perpetuate optimal life. This includes a healthy spine and the freedom from drugs and illness it could provide. To ensure this freedom, it is vital our children are encouraged and taught to adopt their own wellness attitude. Children are very receptive to chiropractic care.

I believe that all members of our society, young or old, can benefit from having a chiropractor on their health team.

"The doctor of the future will give no medicine but will interest the patient in the care of the human frame, and in the cause and prevention of disease.
– Thomas Edison

The secret is out. The doctor of the future is here. Chiropractic is leading the wellness revolution of millions around the world who, under regular chiropractic care, are living life to its fullest. Join us today.

Dr. Amy Michelle Willcockson, D.C.
Chiropractic First, P.A.
Long Lake, MN
952-476-2260
drwchiropracticfirst@netzero.net

Dr. Willcockson specializes in chiropractic biophysics and lifetime family wellness.

PART EIGHT

HEALTHY SPINE = OPTIMAL HEALTH

❧

By Dr. Steven Thiele, D.C.

Do you remember your parents telling you to stand up straight? Well, as usual, they were giving you great advice. As it turns out, standing up straight does much more than even our parents knew about. It makes us look better and more confident. It could also make us feel better by providing more of the energy we need to live life to its fullest.

There is much more to good posture than people realize. Posture is the position of ligaments, muscles and spinal bones. It could directly affect how we feel both immediately and long-term.

To obtain and maintain the best posture, your spine must be in optimal health. This means, looking from the back, your spine should be perfectly straight with each of your 24 spinal bones stacked precisely on top of each other. From a side view, you should see three curves or arcs in your spine. In nature, an arch offers one of the strongest defenses against destructive forces such as gravity and motion.

To achieve a healthy spine, you must first understand what could make your spine unhealthy. The culprits of an unhealthy spine could be emotional, mental or physical stress — all of which could cause your spine to become out of balance.

When your body experiences emotional, mental or physical

stress, your body's inner wisdom strives to adapt and change. The body's defense mechanisms maintain the high level of resistance you need.

Unfortunately, these stresses could overwhelm your body and its natural defenses. This could result in a shift of your spine. Even though you may not feel it, this shifting of your spine could cause a lot of health problems – some immediately painful, some not.

This spinal shifting results in an abnormal vertebral bone structure. This is what chiropractors refer to as subluxation. This spinal imbalance, in which one or more bones may have shifted out of position, could cause areas of your spine to work harder in order to compensate for the area or areas out of balance. This could prompt some very unpleasant results.

The spine consists of 33 bones that interlock with each other. Only the top 24 bones are movable with the vertebrae of the sacrum and coccyx being fused. The vertebrae house nerves that transmit important messages from your brain to your body's organs, tissues and cells. Much like you would expect, your body could suffer when these messages are not transmitting properly.

When the vertebrae are subluxated, the important nerve pathways could become completely blocked resulting in life energy not flowing through the nerve being choked. Not only could this lower your body's resistance, it could also interfere with your body's ability to heal itself. This may leave you fighting off unwanted illnesses and injuries virtually defenseless.

If this condition is not corrected, your body's organs and glands could also be in danger. The organs may not function properly and could cause abnormal body chemistry, diseases, accelerated deterioration and untimely death! Despite this, there are no warning signs or early symptoms of vertebral subluxation.

Your chiropractor is the weapon you have in the fight against vertebral subluxation. Even so, many people have never visited a chiropractor and are not aware of how much better they could feel everyday by having their spines adjusted.

Understanding Chiropractic Care and How It Could Help You

Chiropractic care is the art and science of gently removing damaging pressure placed on the nervous system by a misaligned spinal column.

Your chiropractic doctor will regularly check your posture and other physical signs that could indicate spinal imbalance and nervous system dysfunction. Your doctor will make corrections with accurate spinal adjustments that could enhance your healing ability, performance and resistance.

I believe lowered resistance is the number one cause of all physical breakdowns. Consider vertebral subluxation as a major cause of lowered resistance in the body. Do you see how your health and well-being could be greatly increased with regular chiropractic care?

I believe to achieve optimal health and well-being, regular chiropractic care should be supplemented with a balanced, healthy diet. This includes good nutrition along with the proper intake of water each and every day. In addition, I recommend a regular exercise program and plenty of rest.

Chiropractic care strives for spinal alignment, resulting in total body health and well-being. As chiropractors, our purpose is to educate and adjust as many families as possible in an effort to obtain optimal health through natural care.

Chiropractic is Scientific

The positive results of chiropractic care on our bodies have been well documented. This could be why we hear of and see many celebrities and professional athletes relying on regular chiropractic care. They understand firsthand that their bodies must perform at optimal levels on a day-to-day basis.

Both scientific and completely natural, chiropractic care is safe. It does not require the use of harmful chemicals, but instead relies on our body's own natural defenses. These defenses, along with a healthy lifestyle, help people achieve optimal health.

When the bones of the spine return to normal position, enhanced nervous system function is restored, painful symptoms can be relieved and the body's natural healing process proceeds.

In fact, maintaining your spine may very well be one of the most significant health investments you could make.

Beginning at birth, the spine requires regular maintenance for optimal nerve integrity and optimum health potential. When neglected, spinal misalignment or subluxation could result in tissue and organ dysfunction. Over time, when enough tissue damage or dysfunction occurs, crisis and symptoms result.

Consider this. The famous 19th century French physiologist Claude Bernard and the famous French chemist Louis Pasteur argued throughout their lives as to the cause of disease. Was it the soil or the seed?

Pasteur argued it was the seed (the germ). Bernard argued it was the soil (the body).

These same arguments remain prevalent today. Many medical authors agree germs are certainly a factor in the diseases of man. Others say germs, alone, are not the cause of diseases.

With this in mind, B.J. Palmer, the developer of chiropractic, said, "If the 'germ theory' of disease were correct, there would be no one living to believe it."

As reported at www.chiropracticresearch.org: "Some medical doctors and most chiropractors agree that the germ, though being part of the disease syndrome, is not the direct cause of the disease. First, a person must be susceptible to the germ. The germ will always be with us, and our main concern should be to our resistance to them."

In my opinion, regular spinal adjustments, dietary management and the use of vitamins, minerals and herbal supplementation help to achieve optimal resistance and nerve system function. In addition, proper weight management, daily aerobic exercise, increased pure water consumption and ongoing chiropractic care also offer sensible alternatives for people looking for natural, drugless approaches to pain relief, health restoration and optimal health.

Learn to appreciate your body and the life force within that controls your body's functions. Keep in mind there is no greater miracle in nature than your body's own ability to heal.

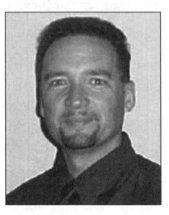

Dr. Steven Thiele, D.C.
Thiele Chiropractic Life Center
Manchester, CT
860-643-8003
www.thielechiropractic.com

CHAPTER SEVEN

THE HEALING OF UNIQUE SUBLUXATIONS

I Trust You, God, But…

❦

By Dr. Joe Henry Rodriguez, D.C.

How do you know if you're healthy? How do you determine if you're not? The standard answer, regardless of where I ask these questions, is "symptoms." That is, if you have any symptoms you could be sick or injured; if you don't have symptoms, you must be healthy.

I believe this kind of thinking is not only dangerous, but could be deadly! Do we live with a symptom-based or reactive philosophy boiling down to "wait until *something* is wrong then react?" Is the usual reaction a pill, potion, shot or surgery?

In my opinion, this is how our health care system is set up, the opposite of the way it could be organized.

Think about this question: When do you get a symptom? Before some sort of damage occurs, or after? Obviously, the answer is AFTER there's been damage.

Today, the two leading causes of death in the United States are heart disease and cancer. Both could be in the body for months, maybe even years, before you feel any symptoms. Often, by the time one recognizes something is wrong, it could be too late.

Surprisingly, as reported in the *Journal of the American Medical Association* (*JAMA*), Volume 284, July 26, 2000, the third leading cause of death after heart disease (700,142 deaths per year) and cancer (553,768) is actually iatrogenic error including deaths from unnecessary surgery, medication errors, hospital errors, infections and adverse reaction to medications. These iatrogenic deaths result in anywhere from 225,000 to 284,000 deaths each year.

Could it be that if the disease doesn't kill you, the treatment might?

Real Health

The whole premise of chiropractic is that God made your body with the amazing ability to heal itself.

Automatically and naturally, your body is always striving towards optimal health and healing. Your body's ability to heal is under the direct control of your nerve system — from your brain to your spinal cord through your nerve structure.

Subluxation, or nerve interference, is a misalignment of the bones along the spinal column. When a vertebra is out of alignment, it could reduce the quantity and quality of nerve flow, which in turn, could affect your health. Eventually, you could feel pain, illness or both. Subluxations can be in your spine for years, even decades, before you feel any symptoms at all. Like heart disease and cancer, they can be caught too late to totally heal them.

The purpose of chiropractic is to detect nerve interference (subluxation), correct misalignment and maintain the correction. This could allow your body to function at its God-given potential.

How It Works

The brain controls, coordinates and monitors all functions in your body. The brain is connected to your body via the spinal cord and nerves. God completely encased the brain within the skull for protection, a truly smart design.

The spinal column protects your delicate lifeline or intelligence line. Nerves branch from your spinal cord to every organ and cell, allowing communication with your brain.

How well your body functions could be directly proportionate to the health of your spine. If a subluxation goes undetected, causing a reduction in nerve flow, the organ connected to that nerve could suffer great damage.

Life is expressed through your nerve flow.

> *"And the Lord God formed man of the dust of the ground, and breathed into his nostrils the breath of life; and man became a living soul."*
> – Genesis 2:7 KJV

Are you living at your God-given potential?

Being a chiropractor, I work with the law of life. The power that made the body could also heal the body. I operate by faith, faith that my God can and will heal if He is allowed to do so.

Grostic/Ortho-Spinology

By doing a 3-D analysis, I am able to detect as little as 1/4 degree tilt, rotation or shift in the atlas. This may cause brain stem compression, tension or both. I adjust very specifically and gently to correct this subluxation. I believe the more specific you are with just about anything, the better results you could receive.

People of all ages come to see me with an array of health challenges. Everything from headaches, migraines, seizure disorder, fibromyalgia, fatigue, acid reflux, esophageal spasms, SLE Lupus, sleeping disorder, allergies and bilateral carpel tunnel. Each of these patients with their different conditions and symptoms had one thing in common: subluxations. Once the subluxations were corrected, they experienced a better quality of life.

As doctors of chiropractic, we educate our patients on health

and healing. Our patients now want what we want for them —
optimal health and wellness.

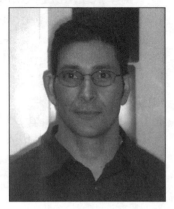

Dr. Joe Henry Rodriguez, D.C.
Shoreline Chiropractic
Austin, TX
512-990-5121
Dr. Rodriquez specializes in
Upper Cervical Chiropractic.

PART TWO

THE EXTREMITY SIDE OF CHIROPRACTIC CARE

By Dr. Patrick C. Andersen, D.C., DABCO

As a youth, I won the Teenage National Power Lifting Championship. I remain active in weight lifting and bodybuilding. I first became interested in chiropractic care at age 17 when I had sustained a back injury during competition. Soon after, I decided to spend my life learning how to help others correct injuries and live pain-free lives through natural chiropractic care.

As I look back over my 25 years of practice and associated training, while new information becomes available, the basic fundamental truth remains constant. Subluxation interferes with the body; while subluxated, it is impossible to be at one's best health.

Other joints within the body can have subluxation, as well as, the classic subluxation of the spine. Extremity subluxations could hinder the progress in the spine.

The right adjustment at the right time in the right place can be life changing.

Many chiropractors use extremity adjusting to help patients see reliable and often dramatic results while achieving optimal health. When subluxations are corrected, joint strain can be removed allowing muscle function, strength and motion to improve.

The TMJ or Jaw Joint

At some point in life, a large number of the American population experiences disc displacement in the jaw joint (TMJ). A small disc on top of the jaw joint can become displaced and cause the jaw to open improperly and shift to one side. When subluxation is present, a person could have difficulty opening the mouth wide enough to place three fingers vertically. The TMJ can be subluxated from sport activities or extended periods of having an open mouth, such as a long dental procedure, stress and even yawning.

Often the jaw joint shows no symptoms until a person is under excess stress. Suddenly, the jaw will begin to cause discomfort. The pain from TMJ syndrome can be excruciating and unrelenting. Proper alignment of the jaw joint by a skilled extremity chiropractor can offer amazing relief, often very quickly.

Shoulder

Stability can be an issue with the shoulders, which are the most mobile joints in the body. There are four joints in the shoulder, one at both ends of the clavicle (collarbone), the ball and socket of the shoulder and scapula (shoulder blade). The shoulder is often injured by falls, heavy lifting or sport activities like throwing.

A common injury can occur in the rotator cuff. Four different muscles form the cuff. The most often injured is the muscle which allows the arm to raise upward and outward about 30 degrees. This muscle can become impinged when the ball of the shoulder is jammed upward, pressing against the underside of the shoulder joint, resulting in muscle weakness and limited ability to move the shoulder without discomfort. Chiropractors can decompress the shoulder to improve the muscle strength and range of motion. If uncorrected, impingement could progress to a rotator cuff tear.

AC Joint

Another frequent shoulder injury occurs with the AC joint, which is the outside joint of the clavicle at the top of the shoulder. When injured or subluxated, raising the arm above the shoulder or reaching forward without pain can be difficult. Muscle weakness can be present and tenderness of the joint is common until adjustment of the AC joint is performed, which can restore strength and function.

SC Joint

The SC joint is the inside joint of the clavicle (collarbone), located near the throat. A self-test for subluxation is to look in the mirror, see if each clavicle bone is at equal height or if either side protrudes or is tender. Once the joint is adjusted, uneven height and protrusion often disappears, restoring strength and range of motion. With shoulder conditions, far too often the focus is on the ball and socket, and not the other joints.

Elbow

When the two joints of the elbow are subluxated, this can cause such things as "tennis elbow" at the outside joint and "golfer's elbow" at the inside joint. Elbow subluxation can be caused if you have too tight of a grip while golfing, the wrong size tennis racket or simply overuse your elbow. The result can be weakness of the triceps muscle (located in the back of the arm) and elbow joint tenderness. For optimal performance, keep your elbows well adjusted.

Wrist and Hand

Carpal Tunnel Syndrome (CTS) is a common condition of the wrist and hand. It occurs when the median nerve becomes entrapped. CTS can cause pain, numbness and a weakened grip. The first CTS signs can be dropping things and being unable to squeeze or open a jar. The wrist has eight small bones, several of which can slip and place pressure on the median nerve. A good self-test for CTS is to press your thumb and little finger together and then try to pull apart to rate your level of strength. Special adjustments realign the small wrist bones reducing pain and improving function.

Hip Joint

The hip joint (ball and socket) can subluxate with a forward or backward displacement. This subluxation often goes undetected. Some back problems can actually begin with the hip. With hip subluxation, the leg involved often fatigues easily while standing. This could cause a person to favor his or her good leg.

Knee

The knee is the largest joint in the body. It is responsible for flexing and extending the lower leg. Injury to the large joint of the knee commonly occurs with sports and heavy lifting. The under surface of the knee cap can become rough and grind against the leg bone. The knees are influenced heavily by the pelvis alignment from above and foot subluxations from below.

Feet

If your feet hurt, it seems like everything hurts. Unfortunately, many people wear shoes that are stylish but terribly uncomfortable. The foot has 26 bones which work together to absorb shock, balance the body and propel the body forward while walking. Approximately 90% of foot conditions are related to a problem called *pronation* where the foot or ankle caves or rolls inward. When a person has pronated feet, each step strains the foot and spine due to overuse and poor shock absorption.

When the foot does not push off properly, the muscle at the bottom of the foot is strained. This can cause inflammation of the tendons and connective tissue. Over time, this could result in heel spurs.

Additionally, poor mechanics from pronation could break down the forefoot arch. This can cause a "bunion" where the big toe displaces outward. With specific adjustments to remove subluxations of the feet and a properly fitted shoe insert called an orthotic, custom made by your chiropractor, much relief for chronic foot pain can be achieved.

I never leave my house without wearing orthotics. They make me feel as though I am walking on a cloud. With my feet being properly supported, there is a stable platform for the spine to be at its best.

Extremity adjusting can and often does strongly complement spinal care and allow better results for chiropractic patients. I would encourage anyone with persistent or problematic joint conditions to pursue an evaluation by a chiropractor certified in extremity adjusting.

Dr. Patrick C. Andersen, D.C., DABCO
Chiropractic USA
Madison, WI
608-833-1282
www.chirousamadison.com

Dr. Anderson is the Area Director for Chiropractic USA in Iowa and Wisconsin. Dr. Anderson is board certified in chiropractic orthopedics with additional training and certifications in sports injuries, spinal trauma (whiplash) and extremities. He is one of America's leading extremity adjusting authorities.

PART THREE

A QUESTION OF BALANCE:
THE UNIVERSAL BENEFITS OF UPPER CERVICAL CHIROPRACTIC

❦

By Dr. Jonathan Gould, D.C.

Many people agree a balanced life is a healthy life. But, achieving balance in today's stress-filled, hurry-up world is not always easy.

Many people are turning to a chiropractic procedure called Upper Cervical Chiropractic (UCC). This gentle, specific treatment allows patients to achieve balance naturally by eliminating neurological irritations at the very points where they begin.

UCC concentrates expressly on the upper two vertebrae where the brain and the spinal column come together. This area is called the atlas. The chiropractor's goal is to make certain the atlas is perfectly level so all spinal column bones follow suit and line up in correct positions.

With properly aligned vertebra, information flows unobstructed from the brain through the entire nervous system. This free flow of information could allow patients to experience natural healing in all areas of their bodies including circulation, digestion, respiration, musculature and behavior.

In my opinion, the most remarkable aspect of this care is the relief you could feel on your very first visit. The balanced life you've been dreaming of could be just one appointment away.

Upper Cervical Chiropractic requires state-of-the-art technology to determine the exact angle to apply small and delicate corrections. UCC could be used for a wide range of disorders.

Upper cervical correction of a patient's atlas is clearly visible on X-rays and offers solid proof spinal balance has begun.

First Visit

Here's what to expect on a first visit to an upper cervical chiropractor. Once in the examination room with your doctor, he or she will ask for a complete history of your symptoms. This could include asking you to describe details of prior types of treatments. This information will provide your chiropractor with an understanding of your health challenge. It will also allow your chiropractor to work in concert with your other healthcare providers to design a care plan unique to you.

Next, a series of pictures will be taken with a Laser Aligned X-Ray Machine so your chiropractor can pinpoint the placement of your correction. This step is very important.

Using the information gathered, your chiropractor will make the adjustment to your atlas.

After the adjustment, I ask my patients to rest for a few minutes before jumping up and heading back out into the big, wild world. They may feel results and are ready to go. I ask patients to savor a moment of post-correction peace-and-quiet. This is more than just pleasant; it's a matter of common sense.

An adjustment can create positive changes in your system. Resting allows healing to really take hold, giving your newly aligned spine the best start possible. I recommend patients include periods of relaxation in their lives in order to achieve balance.

Word of Wisdom

For you to achieve wellness in today's turbulent world, strive for balance within your spine, your nervous system and your everyday activities.

Huge benefits can come from a positive mental attitude and adequate rest and nutrition. But, in these days of non-stop anxiety, it is absolutely critical to create balance within your nervous system to protect against routine, crushing stressors. Hassles like traffic jams, 10-hour workdays and juggling a job and family may be shrugged off. Little-by-little, such irritants can chip away at your ability to stand strong and maintain good health.

When you align the spine, you allow the nervous system an opportunity to fully express itself. This could reduce or reverse disease produced by unresolved stress. Some stress-related sicknesses, like headaches or back pain, may be only too familiar to you. Some, like heart disease, may be silently lurking.

The good news is UCC could give you the upper hand providing both natural healing and prevention. Its results are measurable and specific. They can start from the moment you achieve spinal balance and last a lifetime as you continue to keep that balance in check.

UCC Could Work for You

Do you find your posture is frequently off? Is your head often tilted to one side? Does one shoulder or hip rest higher than the other? Do you suffer from dizziness, jaw problems, ringing in the ears or a specific health problem which has not responded well to conventional treatment?

Upper Cervical Chiropractic could work for you. I feel the most secure balance begins in the center of a body and works its way out. With Upper Cervical Chiropractic, you could find that balance and be able to stand straight and strong, no matter what life throws your way.

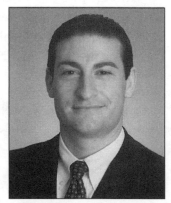

Dr. Jonathan Gould, D.C.
Upper Cervical Chiropractic of New York
White Plains, NY
914-686-6200